Over the Edge and Into the Deep End: Schizophrenia and the Bounds of the Human Mind

OVER THE EDGE AND INTO THE DEEP END:
Schizophrenia and the Bounds of the Human Mind

WRITTEN BY:
Austin Mardon, Catherine Mardon, Lydia Sochan,
Omar Abdul Hadi, Joylen Kingsley, Michaela Dowling,
Shannon Lin, Ann Ping, Vedanshi Vala, Sara Djeddi,
Lilian Yeung, & Romina Tabesh

DESIGNED BY:
Kayla Agustin

2021

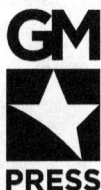

GM
PRESS

First Printing: 2021

Typeset and Cover Design by Kayla Agustin

978-1-77369-654-6

Golden Meteorite Press
103 11919 82 St NW
Edmonton, AB T5B 2W3
www.goldenmeteoritepress.com

CONTENTS

CHAPTER 1

A History of Schizophrenia

Omar Abdul Hadi

Introduction

Schizophrenia is a mental illness that interferes with a person's ability to think clearly, make decisions as well as express and manage emotions (Jablensky, 2010). Today, schizophrenia affects approximately 1% of the world's population (Li et al., 2016). Despite the presence of specific criteria used to diagnose schizophrenia, it still remains as a broad clinical syndrome that is defined by subjective experiences and symptoms (Jablensky, 2010). There are also biological markers that may indicate that one is suffering from schizophrenia, including neurochemical abnormalities, brain dysmorphology and neurocognitive dysfunction (Jablensky, 2010). In addition, schizophrenia is associated with an imbalance of neurotransmitters in the brain (Brisch et al., 2014). The disease is often associated with an increase in dopamine, an increase in the sensitivity of 5HT1A serotonin receptors, a decrease in the sensitivity of 5HT2A serotonin receptors and a decrease in glutamate (NMDA) in the brain (Brisch et al., 2014). There are two types of symptoms for schizophrenia: positive and negative symptoms. Positive symptoms include hallucinations, delusions, paranoia as well as disorganized speech and thinking; in essence, they are symptoms which 'add' to the neurotypical experience. Negative symptoms include social and emotional withdrawal, poor self care, poor judgement, blunted affect and lack of motivation; in other words, these symptoms encapsulate experiences or skills that are 'lacking' from the typical, healthy experience.

How Schizophrenia is Diagnosed

According to the Diagnostic and Statistical Manual of Mental Disorders, 5th edition (DSM-5), a person must exhibit 4 symptoms before a diagnosis in schizophrenia is given (Altschuler, 2001). These criteria are a) continuous disturbance for a period of six months or more, b) the person must exhibit substantial social or occupational dysfunction, c) the person must exhibit at least two of the following five symptoms (delusions, hallucinations, disorganised speech, disorganized or catatonic behaviour or any of the negative symptoms) for a period of 1 month or more, d) general medical history and history of drug misuse or dependence (Altschuler, 2001).

Early Studies on Schizophrenia

The modern concept of schizophrenia was first introduced by German psychiatrist Émil Kraepelin (1856–1927) (Lavretsky et al., 2008). One of the first studies of the neuroanatomical changes (changes in the brain) in schizophrenia was conducted in 1919 by American neurosurgeon Dandy (Lavretsky et al., 2008). Dandy used a technique called pneumoencephalography, a very complex and invasive neurosurgical technique with potentially fatal adverse effects due to the variation in the amount of cerebrospinal fluid (CSF) removed during each procedure (Lavretsky et al., 2008). Using this technique, he showed that patients with schizophrenia show cortical atrophy and ventricular enlargements (enlargement of the four ventricles of the brain) (Lavretsky et al., 2008). Cortical atrophy refers to the gradual degeneration of the outer layer of the brain.

The first study of schizophrenia using magnetic resonance imaging (MRI) was published in 1984 (Lavretsky et al., 2008). MRI studies of the disease consistently show disproportionate volume loss in the temporal lobe and cortical areas, but increased volume of the ventricles (Lavretsky et al., 2008). The first study on schizophrenia using functional magnetic resonance imaging (fMRI) was published in 1991 by Belliveau and colleagues (Lavretsky et al., 2008). fMRI differs from a regular MRI by the images that it produces. An MRI scans anatomy whereas fMRI images metabolic function (Lavertsky et al., 2008). fMRI research in schizophrenia has explored a broad range of cognitive functioning, especially attention, memory, sensory processing, executive function, and psychomotor function (Lavretsky et al., 2008). Both neuroimaging studies using Single Photon Emission Computed Tomography and Positron Emission Tomography (SPECT and PET) have shown three patterns of abnormal cerebral blood flow in schizophrenia (Lavretsky et al., 2008). First, abnormal cerebral blood flow and glucose utilization in the dorsolateral prefrontal cortex (DLPFC) has been linked to impaired working memory and executive function (Lavretsky et al., 2008). Executive functions are cognitive processes that are necessary for behaviour and cognitive control (Lavretsky et al., 2008). Secondly, dysfunction of temporal–limbic circuits have been linked to the manifestation of positive symptoms due to the disinhibition of subcortical dopamine release (Lavretsky et al., 2008). As dopamine D2 receptors are inhibited, essential brain activity may significantly be altered to perceive things that are not reality (Lavretsky et al., 2008). Lastly, positive symptoms such as auditory hallucinations, have been associated with increased blood flow in limbic, medial temporal and subcortical brain areas (Lavretsky et al., 2008). Increased blood flow to these areas of the brain may cause the brain to function well over its normal capacities, leading to symptoms of delusions and hallucinations (Lavertsky et al., 2008)

Today, scientists have been able to deepen their understanding of the pathophysiology of schizophrenia thanks to the advancement of neuroscience and neuroimaging techniques.

Early Studies on Schizophrenia

One of the earliest recorded treatments for schizophrenia is psychosurgery. Also known as neurosurgery for mental disorder (NMD), it was first introduced in the 1880s by Gottlieb Burckhardt (Berrios, 1997). Generally, psychosurgery involves surgically removing or destroying a small portion of the brain (Berrios, 1997). The most common surgery performed was frontal lobotomies, which involves severing some nerve tracts of the frontal lobe, resulting in reduced agitation and impulsive behavior (Lavretsky et al., 2008). This helps to reduce the symptoms of schizophrenia but often simultaneously increases cognitive impairment (Lavretsky et al., 2008). Another type of early schizophrenia treatment commonly used was insulin coma therapy. Insulin coma therapy is a form of psychiatric treatment in which patients are repeatedly injected with large doses of insulin to produce a coma over a period of several weeks (Jones, 2000). It was first introduced in 1927 by psychiatrist Manfred Sakel (Jones, 2000). Insulin coma therapy was widely used between the 1940s and 1950s but it lost popularity due to the discovery of antipsychotic drugs in the 1960s (Jones, 2000).

Modern and Past Drugs Used to Treat Schizophrenia

Today, there are many effective treatments used to relieve the symptoms of schizophrenia. The goal in treatment of schizophrenia is to target symptoms and prevent relapse (Patel et al., 2014). Pharmacotherapy (the use of drugs) is the most typical treatment for schizophrenia but it may lead to adverse side effects and residual symptoms may persist (Patel et al., 2014). Therefore, a mixture of pharmacological and nonpharmacological treatments such as psychotherapy are important for patients with schizophrenia (Patel et al., 2014). It is also crucial to note that nonpharmacological treatments should be used in addition to pharmacotherapy and not as a substitute for them (Patel et al., 2014). There are two types of pharmacological drugs used in the treatment of schizophrenia (Patel et al., 2014). These two types are conventional antipsychotics and atypical antipsychotics. First-generation antipsychotics (FGAs), also known as typical or conventional antipsychotics, work mainly by blocking dopamine receptors (D2) in the brain, which affects the neurotransmission of dopamine by decreasing the activity of dopamine receptors (Patel et al., 2014). Second-generation antipsychotics (SGAs), also known as atypical antipsychotics, affect the neurotransmission of serotonin rather than dopamine (Patel et al., 2014). FGAs are more effective at treating the positive symptoms of schizophrenia than the negative symptoms (Patel et al., 2014).

While the chemical structures of typical antipsychotics are very diverse, almost all share a similar pharmacological effect: the blockage of dopamine D2 receptors in the mesolimbic region of the brain (Li et al., 2016). FGAs can be classified into a number of chemical classes including phenothiazines, thioxanthenes and diphenylbutylpiperidines (Li et al., 2016). Phenothiazines are heterocyclic compounds that contain nitrogen and sulfur groups (Li et al., 2016). Thioxanthenes are structurally related to phenothiazines, their major structural difference being that the nitrogen group in position 10 of phenothiazines is replaced with a carbon atom in thioxanthenes (Li et al., 2016). The first antipsychotic, chlorpromazine, belongs to the phenothiazine family (Li et al., 2016). Today, there are many different FGAs used to treat schizophrenia. Chlorpromazine, perphenazine, fluphenazine, trifluoperazine and levomepromazine are all FGAs that belong to the phenothiazine family (Li et al., 2016). Chlorprothixene, clopenthixol and thiothixene are examples of FGAs that belong to the thioxanthene family. Pimozide, fluspirilene and penfluridol are FGAs that are classified in the diphenylbutylpiperidine class (Li et al., 2016). Despite the availability of many effective FGAs, the most commonly used typical antipsychotic is haloperidol (Li et al., 2016). Haloperidol belongs to a fourth chemical class of FGAs known as butyrophenones (Li et al., 2016). Haloperidol was first synthesized by Bert Hermans in Belgium in February of 1958 and was marketed under the brand name Haldol in Belgium in 1959 (Li et al., 2016). Today, haloperidol is on the World Health Organization's (WHO) list of essential medicines (Li et al., 2016). Haloperidol is the most commonly used FGA because of its preferential binding to dopamine D2 and α1-adrenergic receptors while having negligible affinity for serotonin 5-HT2C, histamine H1 and muscarinic M1 receptors, which are believed to be associated with the adverse effects of FGAs (Li et al., 2016). Although there are many benefits of FGAs, there are also many adverse effects that vary from person to person. These adverse effects include extrapyramidal symptoms, sudden high fever, anticholinergic effects (dry mouth, constipation, urinary retention, bowel obstruction, dilation of pupils, blurred vision and increased heart rate), sedation, skin reactions and orthostatic hypotension (Li et al., 2016). Extrapyramidal symptoms (EPS) are movement disorders that resemble the symptoms of Parkinson's disease. EPS are a result of the blockage of dopamine D2 receptors and they result in four types of symptoms (Li et al., 2016). The first of the four symptoms is acute dystonia which is the involuntary spasm of the muscles in the face, tongue, back or neck (Li et al., 2016). Secondly, EPS can result in bradykinesia which results in rigidity, mask-like faces and stooped posture (Li et al., 2016). Thirdly, EPS also results in akathesia which is pacing, squirming and the desire to constantly be in motion (Li et al., 2016). Finally EPS can result in tardive dyskinesia which results in involuntary twisting and writhing of the face and tongue (Li et al., 2016).

Unlike FGAs, SGAs act on serotonin receptors in the brain, specifically 5-HT2A receptors (Li et al., 2016). Compared to FGAs, SGAs have the same efficacy against positive symptoms of schizophrenia, but a much lower risk of developing extrapyramidal symptoms due to their low affinity towards dopamine D2 receptors (Li et al., 2016). SGAs also have a greater efficacy against the negative symptoms of schizophrenia (Patel et al., 2014). Adverse reactions of SGAs include sedation, orthostatic hypotension, weight gain, risk of developing type II diabetes and anticholinergic effects (drugs that block the action of the neurotransmitter acetylcholine) (Li et al., 2016). Clozapine is one of the most commonly used SGA today. Clozapine has been shown to have antipsychotic effects in humans with a significantly reduced risk of EPS at effective doses (Li et al., 2016). Many SGAs have been developed based on clozapine including risperidone, olanzapine, quetiapine, paliperidone, ziprasidone, lurasidone and sertindole (Li et al., 2016). Clozapine was developed by the Swiss drug company Sandoz in 1961 and was marketed across Europe during the 1970s (Li et al., 2016). Clozapine was a very popular choice for healthcare professionals to choose because of its very rich pharmacological and therapeutic efficacy in treating schizophrenia. Clozapine targets a very broad range of receptors including adrenergic, histaminergic, muscarinic, dopaminergic and serotonergic receptors (Li et al., 2016). Although clozapine is arguably one of the most effective antipsychotic drugs, it was withdrawn from markets due to increased instances of myocarditis (inflammation of the heart muscle), seizures and clozapine-induced agranulocytosis (extremely low granulocytes in the blood) (Li et al., 2016). It was later reintroduced into the US markets in the 1990s strictly for very advanced and treatment-resistant schizophrenia (Li et al., 2016).

Another type of SGA is risperidone. Risperidone has very potent dopaminergic D2 and serotonergic 5-HT2A antagonistic activities (Li et al., 2016). Risperidone was developed by the company Janssen-Cilag between 1988-1992 (Li et al., 2016). It was approved by the Food and Drug Administration (FDA) in 1993 as a treatment for schizophrenia in adults (Li et al., 2016). Aripiprazole is a relatively new antipsychotic representing a third class of SGAs (Li et al., 2016). Unlike clozapine and risperidone, aripiprazole is a pure antagonist of D2 and 5-HT2A receptors (Li et al., 2016). It also acts as a partial agonist for 5HT1A receptors (Li et al., 2016). Brexpiprazole is an analog of aripiprazole that was approved by the FDA in 2015 as a treatment for schizophrenia in adults as well as a treatment for major depressive disorder (MDD) (Li et al., 2016).

The newest antipsychotic drug today is lumateperone (ITI-007) which was approved by the FDA in 2019 (Li et al., 2016). ITI-007 uses a new approach in the treatment of schizophrenia. It acts by targeting multiple neurotransmitter systems at once (Li et al., 2016). ITI-007 also has dual properties, acting as a postsynaptic antagonist and as a pre-synaptic partial agonist of dopamine D2 receptors at the same time (Li et al., 2016). This means that ITI-007 can have inhibitory and excitatory properties (Li et al., 2016). ITI-007 has been shown to help relieve both positive and negative symptoms of schizophrenia; it also has reduced side effects such as lower risks of EPS and cardiovascular side effects (Li et al., 2016).

Today, schizophrenia affects approximately 1% of the entire population. It is a very dangerous mental illness that presents itself in many different forms: different patients can experience wildly different symptoms. At a molecular level, schizophrenia is due to a significant increase in dopamine levels and a decrease in glutamate levels in the brain. Patients of schizophrenia may experience positive or negative symptoms or both. Positive symptoms of schizophrenia include hallucinations, paranoia, and delusions, while negative symptoms include social and emotional withdrawal as well as poor judgement. Schizophrenia is well understood today thanks to advances in neuroscience and neuroimaging. Today, schizophrenia is treated using typical and atypical antipsychotics, drugs that help suppress the symptoms of the disease. Before antipsychotics were made available to the public in the 1960s, healthcare professionals treated schizophrenia using other methods, such as psychosurgery and insulin coma therapy. The two types of antipsychotics available in the modern day help to suppress schizophrenia symptoms using different mechanisms of action. Typical or conventional antipsychotics work mainly by blocking the dopamine receptor (D2) in the brain which affects the neurotransmission of dopamine. Second-generation antipsychotics (SGAs), also known as atypical antipsychotics, affect the neurotransmission of serotonin rather than dopamine. Although these drugs are effective in the treatment of schizophrenia, their use has been associated with severe adverse effects. Currently, there are many more antipsychotic drugs in clinical trials that have the goal of treating schizophrenia without the harmful side effects of modern drugs.

CHAPTER 2

The Subjective Experience of Schizophrenia: An Interview with Dr. Austin Mardon

Joylen Kingsley

Introduction

Mental health is simultaneously one of the most discussed topics in society yet also one of the most misunderstood topics. Society has started the discussion on understanding the basics behind mental disorders, but there is a significant lack of input from those who suffer from mental illnesses. Neurotypical people rarely take time to understand what neurodivergent people experience. The stigma surrounding mental disabilities is enough to prevent people from accesing jobs and to minimize their access to experiences that should and can be equal opportunity. At the very core of the problem, stigmatization, and ignorance towards the label of mental illness often strips people of the basic respect they deserve to receive in society.

Such is the experience of Dr. Austin Mardon, a decorated scientist who has proven to the world time and time again that schizophrenia does not equate to a life without prospects. This chapter explores Dr. Mardon's journey through life as he overcame the societal stereotypes of schizophrenia and how he approached his diagnosis through life. Dr. Mardon grew up in a time where mental health was not discussed, there was a severe lack of resources and medication for mental disorders. Since his diagnosis, Dr. Mardon has shown society that as science develops, so too should social equality.

A Timeline of Dr. Mardon's Experience with Schizophrenia

Dr. Mardon was born in 1962 and showed prodromal characteristics as early as the late 1960s to the early 1970s. Prodromal characteristics refer to precursor symptoms usually to a chronic neurological disorder, as is the case with schizophrenia (George et al., 2017). The concept of prodromal symptoms was introduced in 1911 by Bleuler, and studies show that early medical intervention when prodromal symptoms are present allows for a better prognosis (George et al., 2017). Unfortunately, when Dr. Mardon started presenting prodromal characteristics, medication was not yet widely used. Chlorpromazine, one of the first antipsychotic class medications, had just been introduced in 1952 (Carpenter & Koenig, 2008). Dr. Mardon's main form of treatment was through a child psychiatrist, who suspected he had schizophrenia before his initial diagnosis, speculation was further solidified, as Dr. Mardon's mother developed schizophrenia in 1969. Schizophrenia has an estimated 80% hereditary rate and tends to develop and present itself earlier in males than in females (Trifu et al., 2020).

Dr. Mardon was officially diagnosed in 1985 after graduating from the University of Lethbridge, where he experienced his first episodes of psychosis. Schizophrenia diagnostic criteria can be classified into three categories: positive symptoms, transient psychotic symptoms and genetic risk characterized by functional changes (George et al., 2017). Positive symptoms refer to a distortion of reality, such as hallucination and voices (Carpenter & Koenig, 2008; George et al., 2017). Transient psychotic symptoms refer to temporary but frequent symptoms that are experienced by patients and usually self-resolved within a week (Carpenter & Koenig, 2008; George et al., 2017). Category three or genetic risks are considered in diagnosis if an immediate relative has or had schizophrenia, and the patient has experienced functional decline within the last year (Carpenter & Koenig, 2008; George et al., 2017). Despite his well adjusted lifestyle, Dr. Mardon did not always accept his initial diagnosis. He experienced positive symptoms including voices and hallucinations, but ignored them to the best of his ability. True to his scientific roots, Dr. Mardon braved on, through both graduate school, as well as through multiple expeditions, including to the Antarctic. He describes that particular expedition as successful both on the academic and mental health front, as he was relatively unscathed by his symptoms, but unfortunately he did suffer lung damage from overexposure to the harsh Antarctic climate.

It was after his return from an expedition to the Soviet Union that he experienced a full nervous collapse. The major difference between this incident and the previous nervous episodes, was that for the first time he was unable to hide the extent of his suffering. The collapse resulted in a loss of almost 50 IQ points, and considering his remarkable success as an astronomical scientist, the seeming end of his career. Although life was initially difficult, Dr. Mardon prevailed, he was entered into the Assured Income for the Severely Handicapped program, which provides funding for those with physical and mental disabilities, and he was introduced to medication. He spent much of his time in publishing, starting originally with his father's works and transitioning into his own. Despite his successes Dr. Mardon has had his setbacks including his divorce in the late 1990s, but he serves as a notable example for perseverance, as he has overcome his tribulation time and time again. In 2006, he married his current wife Catherine Mardon, and in 2007 was awarded the Order of Canada, which is one of the greatest academic achievements in Canada. Since then, Dr. Mardon has continued to acquire countless accolades and is one of the most, if not the most decorated individuals in the world with schizophrenia.

Journey Through Presenting Symptoms and Diagnosis

Dr. Mardon's family was already sensitized to schizophrenia because of his mother who was diagnosed in 1969. Therefore, they knew what signs to expect, and Dr. Mardon's father actually suspected that Dr. Mardon had the illness early in his childhood. His suspicions were later confirmed in 1985 with a schizophrenia diagnosis. Dr. Mardon's child psychiatrist suggested that a personal stressor in the 1980s had caused a personality change, and because his schizophrenia had slow onset, Dr. Mardon had no choice but to struggle along. Much like any other disease, symptoms of schizophrenia often vary from person to person, but there are several consistent factors leading to diagnosis. There are three main categories of symptoms associated with schizophrenia: positive symptoms, negative symptoms, and cognitive impairment. Positive symptoms refer to the creation of delusions and hallucinations, as well as generalized disorganization, both in speech and lifestyle (Bassett et al., 1993; Trifu et al., 2020). For Dr. Mardon, positive symptoms manifested in the form of voices and paranoid hallucinations. Negative symptoms are the second category of symptoms and can be further divided into two subsections: a lack of enthusiasm and diminished expression (Trifu et al., 2020). Finally, cognitive impairment prevents individuals from remembering information, learning, and concentrating (Bassett et al., 1993; Trifu et al., 2020). Dr. Mardon experienced all three categories, and even described occasions where his symptoms were overwhelming to the point of him getting lost within his own neighborhood. It was a very dark time for him after his total psychotic break, he considers himself lucky to not have committed suicide.

It took him seven years to finally accept his diagnosis. He was able to hide his symptoms fairly well until the early 1990s when he experienced his full blown nervous collapse. Dr. Mardon went from ignoring his condition to very quickly having to accept the truth, but regardless his desire remained to "keep trying to make it." At the height of his disorder in the early 1990s he came to the difficult decision to "just give up": he figured that he would live on the Assured Income for the Severely Handicapped for the rest of his life. Of course, this decision was not due to a lack of perseverance, but because the job opportunities for persons with mental illnesses were very scarce. Once a person is labeled as disabled, particularly as mentally disabled, systemic discrimination in the workplace limits their job options; it was virtually impossible to work even menial jobs. Dr. Mardon's solution was to keep writing as much as he could, and to volunteer. In his own words, "I couldn't hold a job down, but I could actively volunteer". Dr Mardon's perspective changed when he entered into the Assured Income for the Severely Handicapped program, he realized that he could live comfortably by relying on the provided income. Unlike many others he did not try to exit the program but used the funding to develop himself with the support of the Albertan government. The priority for him was to minimize stressors and to maintain his health.

Dr. Mardon's Experience with Advocacy and Schooling

The Order of Canada in 2007, the Flag of Hope Award in 2001 and the Distinguished Alumni Award of the University of Lethbridge in 2002 are just a few of the awards that Dr. Mardon has accumulated in his life of education and advocacy. By no means was his journey to success considered easy: Dr. Mardon failed many graduate programs, not because of his inability to do the work, but heavily due to barriers caused by the label of schizophrenia. Timing, accommodation, and financial troubles plagued him during his education. It took him a considerable amount of time to complete his postgraduate studies. Dr. Mardon spent almost eight years completing his PhD through distance learning, which in and of itself was a stressor to his disorder. When Dr. Mardon was pursuing his education, disability accommodations were also non-existent, he even remembers having guidance counselors laugh in his face. Although both time and accommodations were significant barriers, Dr. Mardon cited financial troubles as "the biggest barrier" to his education. It is a significant motivator behind his drive to help support students financially, both through scholarships and advice. Again, despite these barriers, Dr. Mardon has succeeded and has even been named a Specially Elected Fellow, by the Royal Society of Canada. He expressed the irony of the situation, as he had failed and been restricted often throughout his education but was still the recipient of one of the highest academic achievements in Canada.

Experience with Medication and Therapeutics

Antipsychotic medication was introduced in 1952, and pharmaceutical research has only been improving in the past few decades (Carpenter & Koenig, 2008). Schizophrenia has a lifelong prevalence, with symptomatic patterns of recurrence and remission. Pharmacotherapy is deemed the leading treatment in reducing positive symptoms and minimizing relapses (Carpenter & Koenig, 2008). Initially antihypertensive drugs were used to reduce dopamine release, as schizophrenia is associated with overstimulation and overproduction of dopamine (Carpenter & Koenig, 2008; Frese et al., 2009). The success of the drug mechanism prompted the creation of chlorpromazine in 1952, and since then about 50 more antipsychotics have entered the market, the majority being antagonists of the D2 dopamine receptors (Carpenter & Koenig, 2008).

Regardless of improvements in pharmacotherapies, at the time of Dr. Mardon's diagnosis, drug therapy for schizophrenia was not common. Initially, Dr. Mardon was in both personal and group therapy with others who struggle with schizophrenia. His psychiatrists encouraged his writing and publications, while suggesting that he accept the help given by the Assured Income for the Severely Handicapped program. His psychiatrist played a significant role in encouraging his work with schizophrenic support groups. Even without medication, he stated that group therapy was remarkably effective, and that he is still in contact with many of the people he met during those therapy sessions.

Dr. Mardon is known for his advocacy of pharmacotherapeutics in schizophrenia, he started medication in the late 1990s and has continued the regimen without fail. Approximately 75% of people with schizophrenia stop taking their medication within the first 18 months (Dobber et al., 2018). Dr. Mardon has been taking his medication consistently for almost 30 years. The population of people who have been on antipsychotics for such an extended period is low, therefore his medication is frequently adjusted. Dr. Mardon has observed that doctors notice his compliance, and are tempted to lower his dosage: they equate his compliance with improvement. Unfortunately, that is not the case, he is still sick, and reducing his dosage has affected him negatively in the past. Of course, antipsychotics have been known to have side effects including increased risk of movement disorders, sedation, and weight gain, but Dr. Mardon's advice is to "just punch through it" (Dobber et al., 2018). He states that "people today do not know how lucky they are, and that the earlier medication was terrible, the only real option for a good prognosis is to take the medication". Dr. Mardon's advice to promote medication is honesty, he encourages discussion on medication, including both the benefits and downfalls, but most importantly he encourages conversation where and when possible.

Dr. Mardon's Personal Experience with Stigmatization and Improvement

Stigmatization of any mental health disorder is a prevalent topic in society, but patients with schizophrenia in particular struggle heavily with the false narrative, painted by stereotypes. Society has a tendency to equate schizophrenia with danger and incompetence, without understanding the nuances of the disease. How can professionals expect people with schizophrenia to cooperate with medication and therapy if society constantly tells them that they are monsters? When patients take their medication, they are considered outsiders, but without their medication, patients risk their health; unfortunately with society's input, many patients would rather die than take antipsychotics to improve their health and condition of life. Alongside his views on stigmatization, Dr. Mardon also emphasized the importance of his providers: while his late psychiatrist was instrumental, the negative reaction from some of his own providers have left lasting impacts.

Unfortunately, the stigmatization was not limited to his care providers; Dr. Mardon also experienced discrimination from his own family for his disorder. After he was diagnosed, his immediate family began to blame each other for Dr. Mardon's schizophrenia. Many of his extended family members also broke off contact because of the shame and stigma. His mother reacted negatively when Dr. Mardon was awarded the Order of Canada, because it seemed like he was publicizing something that he should have hidden in shame. While Dr. Mardon's advocacy for schizophrenia was not well received at home, it provided many opportunities for the general schizophrenia patient population. Much of Dr. Mardon's social support came in the form of his therapy groups, where he received support from those whom he refers to as "unsung heroes".

These support groups actually played an instrumental role in Dr. Mardon's advocacy work. They encouraged him to participate in leadership roles because of his education, and much of his inspiration was drawn from the individuals he interacted with in group settings. In his words, "I kept meeting all these people who were cast out of society, that everyone was ashamed of, all because they were different; they were not lesser human beings, they just had limitations". Dr. Mardon emphasized that it was the discrimination as opposed to the illness itself that is difficult with schizophrenia. He predicts that less discrimination may even encourage more individuals to willingly continue their medication. He observed groups of people who were rejected by their families, and society, and decided to make his own family of the homeless, the mentally ill, the directors of NGOs, and hospital directors. He continued in charity work to provide an equal platform, where the affected could work alongside those with the power to inspire change. He built himself up slowly through the media via his advocacy, and cited that his path was a marathon, not a sprint: advocacy takes time to develop.

When asked about the stigma of mental health in the current generation, Dr. Mardon acknowledges the improvement, and that people are more likely to openly discuss their experiences. Mardon's reception of the Order of Canada was due to his willingness to discuss his experience with schizophrenia when it was a heavily restricted topic. Although Dr. Mardon does fear that open discussion has removed some of the self-responsibility among patients, who abuse understanding, as an excuse to avoid their medication, he believes that discussion is the best way to create a more understanding and tolerant society. His own recommendations to improve the stigma includes advice from his wife: Catherine Mardon. She emphasizes that society should learn to separate the disability from the person, and to realize that patients with mental illnesses are still people. Dr. Mardon himself also suggests that stability and security are the ideal conditions that society can provide for those with schizophrenia. People must be educated to escape poverty, a difficult task when faced with negative labels. Stability, and security in education and the workplace creates positive change towards the perception of patients with schizophrenia.

Conclusion

When Dr. Mardon was initially diagnosed, he felt as though there was no hope. He felt as if he had been given a death sentence, but his mindset has drastically improved. As times have progressed both in his own journey and technologically, he has realized that there is hope and that patients with schizophrenia can function with proper medication and treatment. Patients must choose to take their medication and choose to commit to getting better. Dr. Mardon states that many homeless people who struggle with schizophrenia made the conscious decision to not cooperate when they were sane, but when people relapse into psychotic episodes, it is difficult for them to make informed choices and it is difficult to help those people get healthy again. Dr. Mardon recommends that people put their health first, take their medication, and minimize stress where possible.

In the 36 years since his diagnosis, Dr. Mardon has truly come a long way. He has become an advocate for antipsychotics, a decorated scientist, a mentor, and a philanthropist, but what he cites as the biggest change and advantage to his success is his mindset. He has a sense of purpose in life, a reason to get up in the morning, and a reason to continue his medication regimen. His motivating mindset was not always present, it developed along the way. Dr. Mardon is proof that individuals are not the sum of their illnesses: he is successful despite his schizophrenia, and we must use his life as a testament to the heights one can reach when properly motivated and given the opportunity.

CHAPTER 3

Neurochemical Models of Schizophrenia

Michaela Dowling)

An Introduction

The neuroscience, or more broadly neurobiology, discipline represents the col-
laborative integration of multiple scientific fields, all in pursuit of determining the
intricate specificities within our nervous system (Robertson & Dinsdale, 1972).
Since its origin, specialists in the disciplines of biochemistry, physiology, and
virology have each made advances in the identification of neurodevelopmental
stages, healthy neurological functioning, and the roots of neurologic disease
(Robertson & Dinsdale, 1972).

Of particular interest to neuroscientists is the ability to pinpoint the dysfunction
of specific anatomic structures to identify the causes of certain physiological
symptoms or behavioral abnormalities (Robertson & Dinsdale, 1972). For
instance, lesions to the frontal lobe, the most anterior of the four lobes, has been
correlated with a decrease in conscientiousness in behavior, abnormal grasp
reflexes, and limited control of urination, among other symptoms (Robertson
& Dinsdale, 1972). As such, for patients exhibiting these symptoms, dysfunction
in the frontal lobe region is often of high suspect (Robertson & Dinsdale, 1972).
Nonetheless, as of current, a comprehensive understanding of the functions of
each neurological anatomic structure remains unknown (Robertson & Dinsdale,
1972). Consequently, due to this lack of information, both the diagnoses and
treatments of many neurologic conditions, such as schizophrenia, have not yet
been fine-tuned.

The Nervous System's Functional Unit: The Neuron

Behavior, both normal and abnormal, is the product of the nervous system's
functioning (Hancock & McKim, 2018). As such, it is important to establish the
neurophysiological aspects apparent in the normal functioning of the nervous
system to be able to understand the cause behind dysfunction (Hancock &
McKim, 2018). In general, the nervous system is composed of two primary
cell types: neurons and glial cells (or glia) (Hancock & McKim, 2018). In the
brain, neurons and glial cells are found at nearly equal proportions with a total

of approximately 100 billion each (Hancock & McKim, 2018). Neurons are excitable cells that represent the fundamental unit of the nervous system (Hancock & McKim, 2018). Their function involves the transmission and integration of sensory information to produce an appropriate response (Hancock & McKim, 2018). Previously thought of as secondary to neurons, the function of glial cells has recently become a point of interest for many neuroscientists (Hancock & McKim, 2018). Historically, researchers believed glial cells to serve solely as structural support for neuronal circuits; however, present-day, the function of glial cells has now been attributed to fulfill many other purposes (Hancock & McKim, 2018). For instance, glial cells appear to play a role in the neuron protection, proper metabolic regulation of neurons, and the regulation of neuronal communication (Hancock & McKim, 2018). In conjunction, both neurons and glial cells are vital for the proper functioning of the nervous system (Hancock & McKim, 2018).

A neuron contains three main components: a soma, also called the perikaryon, the dendrites, and an axon (Hancock & McKim, 2018). One exception to this generalization are sensory neurons which do not possess dendrites (Hancock & McKim, 2018). The soma of the neuron ranges in size from 5 μm to 100 μm and contains the organelles essential for neuronal metabolism and upkeep (i.e. mitochondria, nucleus, rough endoplasmic reticulum, Golgi apparatus, etc) (Hancock & McKim, 2018). The axon, stabilized by microtubules and microfilaments, extends an average length of 0.1 μm to 10 μm, with enlarged termini, directly from the soma (Hancock & McKim, 2018). Later, further discussion of axons will be provided in relation to neurotransmitters (NTs) and the propagation of action potentials (Hancock & McKim, 2018). Finally, dendrites are shorter projections located on the opposite side of the soma from the axon (Hancock & McKim, 2018). These projections are involved in the reception of signals from neighbouring neurons (Hancock & McKim, 2018). As such, to satisfy this role, dendrites contain neurotransmitter receptors at their termini (Hancock & McKim, 2018).

Neurotransmitters and Action Potentials

To initiate appropriate responses to the ever-changing environmental conditions an organism is exposed to, its neurons must be in constant communication (Hancock & McKim, 2018). As a result, our nervous system has evolved to become capable of both efficient and effective transmission of information throughout the body (Hancock & McKim, 2018). It is important to note that the neurophysiology of the nervous system and neurotransmitter involvement is complex and broad (Hancock & McKim, 2018). Consequently, this section will only be providing a brief introduction of neurophysiological topics on which the discussion of schizophrenia will be constructed.

In comparison to the inside of a neuron, the outside of the neuron is relatively negative (Hancock & McKim, 2018). Consequent to the uneven localization of three main ions (i.e. K+, Na+, and Cl-) this potential difference, termed the resting membrane potential, most commonly falls around -70 millivolts (mV) (Hancock & McKim, 2018). While Na+ and Cl- are more highly concentrated on the exterior of the neuron, K+ is found at higher concentrations in the neuron's interior (Hancock & McKim, 2018). When a neuron becomes stimulated and surpasses its threshold of excitation, Na+ channels open allowing the interior of the cell to become more positively charged (Hancock & McKim, 2018). This process is defined as depolarization (Hancock & McKim, 2018). As more Na+ passes into the cell, K+ channels also open, allowing K+ to exit the cell due to their concentration gradient and the positive charge of the cell's interior (Hancock & McKim, 2018). Upon reaching a membrane potential of approximately +40mV, Na+ channels close (Hancock & McKim, 2018). As K+ continuously leaves the cell, the neuron's membrane potential begins to return to its resting potential (Hancock & McKim, 2018). This phase is known as the repolarization of the neuron (Hancock & McKim, 2018). As K+ channels are slow to close, the neuron briefly enters a period of having a more negative charge in its interior than found during its resting potential, resulting in the neuron's hyperpolarization (Hancock & McKim, 2018). After a brief period, the sodium potassium pumps found within the membrane allow for the return of the resting membrane potential (Hancock & McKim, 2018). All together, the depolarization, repolarization, and hyperpolarization of the neuron's membrane is known as an action potential (Hancock & McKim, 2018). It is important to note that upon influx, the Na+ ions migrate horizontally through the neuron (Hancock & McKim, 2018). This allows for the propagation of the action potential along the neuron's membrane as different sections reach their threshold of excitation (Hancock & McKim, 2018).

However, to allow for the propagation of the action potential between neurons, a different mechanism must occur (Hancock & McKim, 2018). Neurons communicate with one another across a specialized gap known as the synaptic cleft within a synapse (Hancock & McKim, 2018). The synapse is responsible for connecting the terminal buttons of a cell (presynaptic neuron) to another cell (postsynaptic neuron) (Hancock & McKim, 2018). As an action potential migrates horizontally across the membrane of a neuron it eventually reaches the neuron's terminal button (Hancock & McKim, 2018). This location is populated with spherical structures named synaptic vesicles which contain chemicals called neurotransmitters (Hancock & McKim, 2018). As the incoming action potential stimulates the neuron's terminal button, voltage-gated calcium (Ca2+) channels open, in turn, causing an influx of Ca2+ (Hancock & McKim, 2018). These ions promote the fusion of the synaptic vesicles with the neuron's membrane, inducing the exocytosis of neurotransmitters into the synaptic cleft (Hancock & McKim, 2018). Crossing the synaptic cleft, the released neurotransmitters reach the postsynaptic neurons where they interact with their appropriate receptor (Hancock & McKim, 2018). Upon binding, the neurotransmitter can induce a variety of mechanisms or voltage-gated channels depending on its bound receptor. In this way, action potentials are transmitted between neurons (Hancock & McKim, 2018).

The Two Dopamine (DA) Hypotheses: The DA Hypothesis of Schizophrenia and the DA Imbalance Hypothesis

To begin the discussion of the various neurochemical models of schizophrenia, it is essential to first introduce the identified involvement of dopamine (DA) within the disease. Dopamine is a neurotransmitter known to play a vital role in the regulation of the mesolimbic (reward-seeking) and nigrostriatal (motor response) dopamine systems (Cachope & Cheer, 2014). Within both of these pathways, dopamine has implications on a wide range of forebrain anatomic structures; as such, dopamine up- or down-regulation has been associated with many distinct behaviors (Cachope & Cheer, 2014). Investigations into the irregularities of dopamine synthesis, release, metabolism, and variation of receptor prevalence with regards to schizophrenia have been ongoing within the scientific community (Cachope & Cheer, 2014). The first hypothesis correlating dopamine irregularities to schizophrenia proposed dopamine overreactivity as causative of the positive symptoms of schizophrenia (Andreasen & Flaum, 1991). Positive symptoms of schizophrenia include hallucinations, disorganized thought and speech, as well as delusions (Andreasen & Flaum, 1991). Support for this hypothesis is rooted in the discovery that the mechanism of antipsychotic drugs involves the inhibition of D2 receptors (Andreasen & Flaum, 1991). Furthermore, the ability of dopamine-enhancing drugs to induce a psychosis-like state provides additional support for this postulation (Andreasen & Flaum, 1991).

However, over recent years, physicians and researchers alike have begun to put more emphasis on the negative symptoms characteristic of the schizophrenia diagnosis (Andreasen & Flaum, 1991). Negative symptoms include lack of speech, volition (apathy), the inability to feel pleasure (anhedonia), withdrawal from social settings, and affect flattening (Andreasen & Flaum, 1991). Interestingly, in contrast to the positive symptoms, negative symptoms are not resolved by the D2-antagonist drugs (Andreasen & Flaum, 1991). This finding prompted the reform of the original dopamine hypothesis to create the dopamine imbalance hypothesis (Meyer & Quenzer, 2019). As with the original dopamine hypothesis of schizophrenia, this hypothesis postulates that the hyperactivity of dopamine within the mesolimbic pathway (reward pathway) is responsible for the onset of schizophrenia's positive symptoms (Meyer & Quenzer, 2019). However, extending on this original hypothesis, proponents of the novel hypothesis indicate that the lack of dopamine is causative of many of the negative symptoms associated with schizophrenia (Meyer & Quenzer, 2019). Specifically, negative symptoms have been traced to the lack of dopamine transmission to the D1 receptors mesocortical pathway, which is responsible for motor responses (Meyer & Quenzer, 2019).

The Neurodevelopmental Model

The proposal of the neurodevelopmental model represents the combination of anatomical and neurochemical irregularities found within patients with schizophrenia (Meyer & Quenzer, 2019). Patients with schizophrenia often display characteristic anatomical changes in their brains (Meyer & Quenzer, 2019). Using both computerized tomography (CT) and magnetic resonance imaging (MRI), atrophy (degeneration) of the prefrontal and temporal lobes, basal ganglia, and limbic regions, among other structures, has been identified (Meyer & Quenzer, 2019). Furthermore, studies involving positron emission tomography (PET) and single-photon emission computerized tomography (SPECT) demonstrate that individuals with schizophrenia tend to have less blood flow to their prefrontal cortex (PFC) in cognitively-demanding tasks as compared to healthy controls (Meyer & Quenzer, 2019). The decline in PFC functioning is termed hypofrontality and is strongly correlated to the reduction of executive functioning, working memory, problem solving, and response inhibition (Meyer & Quenzer, 2019). As such, the neurodevelopmental model of memory postulates that the negative symptoms of schizophrenia are implications of hypofrontality (Meyer & Quenzer, 2019).

This hypothesis is further supported through two main types of research: lesion studies and animal experimentation (Meyer & Quenzer, 2019). First of all, the neurodevelopmental hypothesis is supported by the similarity of symptoms of those with schizophrenia and studies of those with frontal lobe lesions (Meyer & Quenzer, 2019). Frontal lobe lesion studies include patients suffering from frontal lobe damage or who have undergone a frontal lobotomy (Meyer & Quenzer, 2019). In both patients with frontal lobe lesions and those with schizophrenia, deficits such as inadequate social functioning, emotional blunting, inflexible problem-solving strategies, and amotivation are apparent (Meyer & Quenzer, 2019).

Proponents of this model have additionally relied on findings from animal experiments to support this hypothesis (Meyer & Quenzer, 2019). In animal experimentation, researchers have identified that the injection of D1 receptor antagonists results in the formation of impulsive behaviors (Meyer & Quenzer, 2019). On the other hand, D1 agonists have been associated with the recovery of appropriate cognitive functioning for animals previously treated with a dopamine neurotoxin (Meyer & Quenzer, 2019). These findings indicate the importance of dopamine interacting with the D1 receptor in the maintenance of proper cognitive functioning (Meyer & Quenzer, 2019). In addition, they allude that the downregulation of dopamine in this area may be causative of schizophrenia's negative symptoms (Meyer & Quenzer, 2019). Moreover, this model highlights that the onset of negative systems may be due to the destruction of mesocortical cells within the ventral tegmental area (VTA) located in the frontal lobe (Meyer & Quenzer, 2019). These mesocortical cells are foundational for the creation of a healthy stress response (Meyer & Quenzer, 2019). As such, a decline in their population in the VTA, or their poor development, would result in a patient's inability to respond appropriately to stressful situations, such as in various social settings (Meyer & Quenzer, 2019).

In description of the origin of positive symptoms, the neurodevelopmental model hypothesizes the increased turnover rate of dopamine within the mesolimbic pathway (Howes & Murray, 2014). This is supported by the finding that antipsychotic-induced dopamine receptor blockade pharmaceuticals are effective in the reduction of common positive symptoms (i.e. hallucinations, increased fearfulness, decreased emotional regulation, etc.) (Howes & Murray, 2014). Despite this postulation, the exact cause of the upregulation of dopamine within this pathway has yet to be deduced. Current studies are investigating the possible influence of early-life stressors, such as Cesarean births, which has been correlated to an increase in dopamine concentrations (Howes & Murray, 2014). Nonetheless, as research progresses the neurodevelopmental model continues to be a prevalent model to uncover the foundations of schizophrenia's pathogenesis.

The Glutamate Model

Similar to the dopamine hypothesis, the glutamate model of schizophrenia postulates the abnormal regulation of a neurotransmitter in the formation of symptoms characteristic to schizophrenia (McCutcheon et al., 2020). Glutamate is the most common excitatory neurotransmitter found within the central nervous system, which consists of the brain and the spinal cord (McCutcheon et al., 2020). Upon binding to its appropriate receptor on the postsynaptic neuron, N-methyl D-aspartate (NMDA) in the case of glutamate, an excitatory neurotransmitter increases the probability of an action potential being fired (McCutcheon et al., 2020). As such, the release of glutamate is associated with the propagation of action potentials throughout neural circuits (Hancock & McKim, 2018). In particular, the NMDA receptor has been correlated to contributing towards one's working memory (McCutcheon et al., 2020).

The beginnings of this model originated in experimentation with NMDA antagonists, molecules that inhibit its function, on both healthy patients and those diagnosed with schizophrenia (Egerton et al., 2020). Following treatment with NMDA antagonists, healthy subjects display behaviors mirroring the negative symptoms of schizophrenia (Egerton et al., 2020). Furthermore, individuals with schizophrenia find their current symptoms upregulated upon the treatment (Egerton et al., 2020). This finding primed the current widespread scientific interest in the glutamate's role in schizophrenia (Egerton et al., 2020).

Unlike dopamine, glutamatergic neurons are not localized within select areas of the brain or along designated tracts; on the contrary, they are greatly dispersed (Egerton et al., 2020). As a consequence, the dysfunction of glutamate signalling does not produce an easily identifiable symptom as can be noticed with the postulations of the dopamine hypothesis (Egerton et al., 2020). Building from the initial study, current research indicates the glutamate neurons from the prefrontal cortex are responsible for the activation of the mesocortical neurons (Hancock & McKim, 2018). Therefore, a decrease in glutamate signalling would result in the decrease of dopamine release within the prefrontal cortex of the brain, inducing negative symptoms (Hancock & McKim, 2018). Additionally, low levels of glutamate have been found within the ventral tegmental area (VTA) which are normally utilized to excite GABA neurons (Egerton et al., 2020). These GABA neurons are inhibitory; moreover, they are responsible for the inhibition of dopamine release in the nucleus accumbens (Egerton et al., 2020). Consequently, the irregular high levels of dopamine within the nucleus accumbens due to low glutamate signalling early in this pathway would lead to the positive symptoms (Egerton et al., 2020). In both the onset of the positive and negative symptoms, the involvement of the low levels of glutamate on dopamine regulation is apparent (Egerton et al., 2020).

Final Thoughts

Overall, the neurochemical basis of schizophrenia, while remaining a prominent subject of current scientific research, has provided the scientific community with preliminary answers into the foundational cause of schizophrenic symptoms. As discussed, the role of dopamine, neural anatomic abnormalities, and glutamate, each appear to be associated with the initial onset and progression of the disease (Meyer & Quenzer, 2019). However, as the characteristics of schizophrenia are not uniform, the involvement of each of these may vary among individuals (McCutcheon et al., 2020). For instance, while dysfunction in dopamine pathways may prove significant in one's disease, it may be observed to a lesser extent, or even not at all, in another's (McCutcheon et al., 2020). Nonetheless, the identification of neurochemical and neurobiological abnormalities have provided researchers with a base for the development of pharmaceuticals suitable for treatment of schizophrenia.

CHAPTER 4

The Sociocultural and Environmental Attributes of Schizophrenia

Shannon Lin

Introduction

There is a wealth of evidence that a combination of social, cultural, and environmental factors contribute to the risks of developing schizophrenia (Dein, 2017; Essock, 2017; Fearon & Morgan, 2006; Hooley, 2010; Krabbendam & van Os, 2005; Myers, 2011; van Os & McGuffin, 2003). While there are no direct correlations that deem these factors to cause schizophrenia in and of itself, there are various ways they can make an impact on the development of schizophrenia by exacerbating its risks and its underlying genetic contributions (Krabbendam & van Os, 2005; Myers, 2011; van Os & McGuffin, 2003). Considering the information provided in the previous chapters, the following chapter will discuss the external mechanisms that interact with biological ones to provide an all-around understanding of the causes of schizophrenia. Understanding these risks can assist with identifying the social stressors that lead toward increased incidences of schizophrenia, and the ways that their effects can be mediated (Krabbendam & van Os, 2005; van Os & McGuffin, 2003).

Social Factors Attributed to Schizophrenia

As it is widely understood that social environments are highly influential in determining an individual's mental state, several studies have found a selection of social factors to increase the risks of developing psychotic disorders such as schizophrenia (Hooley, 2010; Myers, 2011; van Os & McGuffin, 2003). Conditions and experiences such as adverse life events, childhood abuse, and exposure to trauma can exacerbate these risks, as well as psychosocial factors including high degrees of daily stress, low socioeconomic status, and cumulative social disadvantages (Myers, 2011; van Os & McGuffin, 2003). Considering that a number of social scientists and clinicians are increasingly convinced that social factors cause schizophrenia, one starts to wonder whether these risk factors can be reduced or prevented through behavioural or environmental changes (van Os & McGuffin, 2003). It has also been found that the social difficulties and deficits that appear early on are similar to those that are presented in later stages of the illness (Hooley, 2010).

While the explanations for the social causes of schizophrenia are varied, there are also a number of social effects that manifest through schizophrenia. Hooley (2010) presents the concept of social competence, which describes "how well a person is doing in day-to-day social situations" (p. 238). At any stage of their illness, those who are diagnosed with schizophrenia, exhibit global difficulties in social competence (Hooley, 2010). As a result, patients with schizophrenia demonstrate weaker verbal and nonverbal skills, perform poorly on social-cognitive tasks, and display difficulties in social problem solving (Bellack et al., 1994, as cited in Hooley, 2010; Hooker & Park, 2002 and Pinkham & Penn, 2006, as cited in Hooley, 2010). From these findings, it must be emphasized that the overall social performance in those with schizophrenia is affected by deficits in a broad range of skill areas as opposed to severe problems in one particular domain (Hooley, 2010). These social impairments are often misunderstood by others who interact with them, which leads to increased negativity, social distance, and rejection by others, and oftentimes creates difficulties for these individuals to fit in with a social world (Hooley, 2010). Their stigmatized status in society has been found to challenge their social functioning even further (Hooley, 2010). One branch of these social interactions that has been found to contribute to increased incidences of schizophrenia is culture, which can be expressed as a social disadvantage by individual-level racism and one's migration status (Fearon & Morgan, 2006; Myers, 2011).

Cultural Factors Attributed to Schizophrenia

For individuals who are ethnic minorities, migrants, and even second-generation immigrants, studies consistently find that these groups experience increased rates of schizophrenia, which suggests that the social context plays a role in the varying stages of the disorder (Fearon & Morgan, 2006; Myers, 2011). The feelings of isolation, fragmentation, and instances of discrimination that occur amongst these populations also plays a role in the higher rates of schizophrenia found within these groups (Fearon & Morgan, 2006; Myers, 2011). This finding of increased social exclusion amongst migrant populations is important in particular, as migrants are more likely to settle in urban centres than rural areas, which results in a greater degree of social adversity experienced when compared to their indigenous counterparts (Fearon & Morgan, 2006; Krabbendam & van Os, 2005). Such experiences may include the migration process, unemployment, low socioeconomic status, and cumulative social disadvantage that are profound in migrant groups (Myers, 2011).

Elevated rates of schizophrenia can also be attributed to the institutionalized racism that exists within host cultures, and individual-level racism that occurs amongst migrant groups due to their structural position in society (Fearon & Morgan, 2006). When considering the demographics of urbanized communities, the rates and risks are increased in areas of "low ethnic density," especially in regions with a low ratio of darker-skinned immigrants compared to lighter-skinned individuals (Myers, 2011, p. 307). For example, Myers (2011) states that from a UK study, Black people who comprise less than 25% of their neighborhood's population have an increased risk of developing schizophrenia by threefold. Other studies find that African Americans are three times more likely than European Americans to be diagnosed with schizophrenia (Myers, 2011). In a study by Fearon and Morgan (2006), this trend toward elevated rates of schizophrenia is found to be evident in second generations of migrants as well. The authors, along with Krabbendam and van Os (2005), stress that when any form of social adversity is experienced for prolonged periods, psychosis may occur, explaining the high rates of psychosis among migrant groups.

Similar to the stigmatizing effects held against individuals with schizophrenia, this can also be found rooted within the beliefs and values of various cultures themselves (Dein, 2017; Myers, 2011). While the rates of schizophrenia are increased in ethnic minority populations, Myers (2011) suggests that the incidences, symptoms, course, and outcomes of the condition are varied across cultural contexts, while Dein (2017) states that cultures attribute the meanings and effects of mental illnesses differently. This is best understood when one considers that the expression of schizophrenia across ethnically diverse populations varies significantly (Dein, 2017). Basic symptoms of schizophrenia such as hallucinations, anhedonia (difficulty or inability to feel and experience pleasure), antisocial behaviour, depressive symptoms, emotional processing deficits (neural regulation of basic or complex emotions), and mood induction (reduced ability to discriminate, experience, and express emotions) are experienced and expressed differently across cultures (Dein, 2017; Habel et al., 2000; Myers, 2011). For example, hallucinations are shaped by local cultural expectations and meanings, which makes them "pathoplastic" (Dein, 2017, p. 64).

Due to these "differing cultural models of reality" that are expressed through experiences of schizophrenia, it is therefore important to be conscious of the cultural relevance of symptoms that are presented in various ethnic groups when diagnosing an illness such as schizophrenia (Dein, 2017, p. 64; Myers, 2011). Symptoms that are deemed to be clinically significant, through this lens, can also be desensitized and be viewed as insignificant as they could be examples of culturally acceptable reactions to trauma, exposure, dissociation, and anxiety (Myers, 2011). As such, each culture also has varying degrees of stigma that is associated with conditions such as schizophrenia, which affects its prognosis and treatment processes (Dein, 2017). A unique finding by Dein (2017) is that schizophrenia has a better prognosis in non-industrialized societies. In 'developing' countries such as Mauritius, Colombia, Nigeria, and India, for example, Dein describes them to have differing expectations and norms regarding employment demands and expression of emotion compared to the United States, which results in lower degrees of stigma. Ultimately, the symptoms and manifestations of schizophrenia vary across different cultures, depending on their norms and degree of sociocentricity (Dein, 2017).

Environmental Factors Attributed to Schizophrenia

Exemplified above, there are several ways that sociocultural factors can interact with each other and impact the risks and vulnerability of developing schizophrenia. In addition to that, extreme social adversities in combination with environmental adversities drastically increase the risk of developing conditions such as schizophrenia (Essock, 2017). This trajectory of undergoing continuous, "repeated environmental insults," has been found to strongly attribute with an individual's vulnerability to the effects of adversity, even in studies that show differing rates of schizophrenia in sociocultural groups that are considered to be genetically similar (Krabbendam & van Os, 2005; Myers, 2011, pp. 305-306; van Os & McGuffin, 2003). For example, Essock (2017) finds that in environments with multiple deprivations, more young people experience schizophrenia. These effects are also profound in disadvantaged neighborhoods, especially for migrants who reside in urban regions that are densely populated (Essock, 2017; Fearon & Morgan, 2006; Krabbendam & van Os, 2005). Within these urban areas, the rate of schizophrenia is double the rate of those in rural areas (Krabbendam & van Os, 2005). All in all, multiple studies have found urbanicity to negatively influence migrant and ethnic minority populations, and increase their risks of schizophrenia (Fearon & Morgan, 2006; Krabbendam & van Os, 2005; van Os & McGuffin, 2003).

Analyzed by Fearon and Morgan (2006), an early American study by Ødegaard (1932) finds that Norweigian migrants to the United States exhibit twice as many cases of schizophrenia when compared with native-born Americans or Norweigians (as cited in Fearon & Morgan, 2006). In the latter studies by Malzberg (1939-1941; 1949-1951) mentioned in the article by Fearon and Morgan, the author states that foreign-born residents of New York State experience higher first-admission rates for schizophrenia (as cited in Fearon & Morgan, 2006). Studies on the post-World War II United Kingdom, which experienced a large influx of migrants from Commonwealth countries such the Caribbean and Indian subcontinent, report rates of schizophrenia higher than the expected amount within the migrant populations of African-Caribbean origin (Fearon & Morgan, 2006). This is stressed in the study by Harrison and colleagues (1997) in Nottingham using epidemiological principles (as cited in Fearon & Morgan, 2006). Precisely, Harrison et al. finds that when compared with the general population in Nottingham, the rate of schizophrenia is increased well over 12-fold in the African-Caribbean community (as cited in Fearon & Morgan, 2006). A minimum of 18 studies on this issue result in similar statistics, where the rates of schizophrenia are elevated in the African-Caribbean population when compared to the White population (Fearon & Morgan, 2006). These inflated rates are also evident in ethnic minority groups (King et al., 1994, as cited in Fearon & Morgan, 2006).

These statistics therefore assume the causality of environmental risk factors for schizophrenia (Krabbendam & van Os, 2005). Ultimately, these findings have established the need to investigate whether the impact of environmental factors correlates with the genetic aetiology (genetic attribution or causation) for psychosis (Krabbendam & van Os, 2005; van Os & McGuffin, 2003). While the risks of schizophrenia can be exacerbated through social stressors and environmental interactions, this effect can also be demonstrated through what is known as the gene-environment interaction, or the genotype-phenotype relationship (Essock, 2017; Krabbendam & van Os, 2005; Myers, 2011; van Os & McGuffin, 2003). The unique aspect about this effect is the bilateral relationship that occurs between this gene-environment interaction (Krabbendam and van Os, 2005). Explained by Krabbendam and van Os (2005), there is an increasing likelihood that the genetic effects in schizophrenia are conditional on the environment and vice versa, where the environmental effects are conditional on genetic risk. In other words, it is possible that the genetic components of schizophrenia occur as a result of environmental impacts, while the environment can also be a response to an individual's genetic risk level of schizophrenia. While the article by van Os and McGuffin (2003) argues that social stressors alone cannot cause schizophrenia, this evidence may suggest that social and environmental factors have the potential to impact individuals who have a genetic predisposition for developing schizophrenia. This indicates that there are steps to reduce or prevent these risk factors through environmental changes (van Os & McGuffin, 2003).

Concluding Thoughts

By exploring the cultural and environmental branches of social interactions, this provides a broader context of research that seeks to identify the causes and risk factors of schizophrenia. Altogether, the research demonstrates the various social, cultural, and environmental impacts that encompasses the comprehensive nature of schizophrenia, which suggests that both social exclusion and environmental deprivations can exacerbate the risks and rates of schizophrenia (Essock, 2017; Fearon & Morgan, 2006; Krabbendam & van Os, 2005; Myers, 2011; van Os & McGuffin, 2003). Most profoundly, the stigma that surrounds individuals with schizophrenia leads to frequent negative encounters of rejection by others (Hooley, 2010).

Additional social challenges that heighten the risks and rates of schizophrenia occur through disadvantages that are prevalent in ethnic minorities and migrant groups (Essock, 2017; Fearon & Morgan, 2006; Krabbendam & van Os, 2005; Myers, 2011; van Os & McGuffin, 2003). Within urban communities that consist of low ethnic density, these populations are found to experience greater bouts of social exclusion alongside institutionalized and individual-level racism, even within their second generation successors (Fearon & Morgan, 2006; Krabbendam & van Os, 2005; Myers, 2011). These factors must be considered in the prognosis of schizophrenia, as well as the cultural variants that view, experience, and express schizophrenia and its symptoms differently (Dein, 2017; Habel et al., 2000; Myers, 2011). Lastly, by considering the genetic components that contribute to the aetiology of schizophrenia, the articles by Essock (2017) Krabbendam and van Os (2005), Myers (2011), and van Os and McGuffin (2003) express that the relationship between the genotype and phenotype can be mediated by the environment through the gene-environment interaction. Finding ways to gain control over these factors is key to reducing the risks and mediating the effects of schizophrenia, especially for individuals with a genetic predisposition for the illness (Krabbendam & van Os, 2005; van Os & McGuffin, 2003). While the causality of schizophrenia through these factors alone is a complex ordeal, taking a comprehensive approach through understanding its social, cultural, and environmental attributes can facilitate feasible ways the condition can be prevented and treated in the future (Krabbendam & van Os, 2005; Myers, 2011; van Os & McGuffin, 2003).

CHAPTER 5

Schizophrenia as a Disorder of Consciousness

Ann Ping

Introduction

Schizophrenia is a complex neuropsychiatric disorder that presents clinical symptoms such as hallucinations, delusions, disorganization of thought, passivity phenomena (phenomena in which one feels like they are under the control of others), disorganized behaviour, and apathy (Giersch & Mishara, 2017; Venkatasubramanian, 2015). It affects more than 1% of the population (Giersch & Mishara, 2017). Additionally, patients with schizophrenia may also exhibit impairments in basic sensory processing and higher cognitive functions (Uhlhaas & Singer, 2010). Despite decades of research, the pathophysiology of schizophrenia is still not completely understood, and there exist many hypotheses regarding the causes of schizophrenia (Uhlhaas & Singer, 2010). However, investigations into the neurophysiological underpinnings of schizophrenia are promising; much of the research indicates that impaired function at a neuronal level may contribute to the psychotic phenomena and cognitive dysfunctions that characterize schizophrenia (Uhlhaas & Singer, 2010).

Two notable models that point to the neuron to explain schizophrenia are the 'disconnection hypothesis' and the 'Orch OR' theory. The disconnection hypothesis proposes that schizophrenia disrupts signalling among brain regions, systems, or cellular circuits (Shin et al., 2011). Neural oscillations (rhythmic electrical activity in the central nervous system) are crucial to the coordination of brain activity. Abnormalities in the synchronization of neural oscillations have been shown to be implicated in schizophrenia (Uhlhaas & Singer, 2010). The Orch OR theory is more controversial and proposes that schizophrenia is a disorder of the consciousness, where consciousness involves quantum processes in the microtubules of neurons (Venkatasubramanian, 2015). This chapter will first review the research on the association between aberrant neural oscillations and schizophrenia, then review the research on the Orch OR theory and its connection to schizophrenia.

How to Detect Neural Oscillations

To preface the discussion on neural oscillations and schizophrenia, it would be useful to understand how neural oscillations, or brain waves, are detected.

Neural oscillatory activity is examined with electroencephalography (EEG) and magnetoencephalography (MEG). The EEG is the record of brain electrical fields, while the MEG is the record of brain magnetic fields (Lopes da Silva, 2013). First, it is worth addressing what exactly a neural oscillation is. When pyramidal neurons, which are a type of neuron found in the cerebral cortex, are activated, intra- and extracellular currents flow (Lopes da Silva, 2013). These currents have a longitudinal (parallel to the axon) and transverse (perpendicular to the axon) component (Lopes da Silva, 2013); the transverse components cancel each other out, resulting in a current along the main axes of the neurons. As the current moves along consecutive neurons, local electrical field potentials and local magnetic fields are generated. The electrical fields are open fields, meaning that they can be detected at a distance from the neuronal source, while the magnetic field lines curl around the neuronal main axis (Lopes da Silva, 2013). These create the EEG and MEG signals, which are described in terms of frequency bands, or 'oscillations'.

Neural synchrony (synchronization of neural oscillations) is reflected in the amplitude of the signals. If neurons fire simultaneously, the rhythmic changes in the electric potential will add up, resulting in a signal of larger amplitude (Musall et al., 2012). Using the EEG and MEG, oscillations of various frequencies can be detected, including delta (0–4 Hz), theta (4–8 Hz), alpha (8–12 Hz), beta (12–30 Hz) and gamma (30–200 Hz) (Williams & Boska, 2010). These different oscillation frequencies are correlated with different cognitive processes, such as consciousness, memory, and attention (Williams & Boska, 2010).

Neural Oscillations and Schizophrenia

In schizophrenia research, gamma oscillations are a major focus. Gamma oscillations are thought to be involved in information transfer between brain regions (Williams & Boska, 2010). In a study on gamma oscillations in the cat visual cortex, it was found that neurons fire at nearly the same time during a cycle of gamma oscillations to simultaneously convey visual information—this indicates that gamma oscillations may serve to 'bind' groups of neurons to convey 'oneness' (Williams & Boska, 2010). Additionally, studies in the prefrontal cortex have shown that gamma oscillations may also be involved in working memory (Williams & Boska, 2010). Working memory allows one to retain information for a short time, and is used in the execution of cognitive tasks such as decision-making and reasoning. In fact, the amplitude of gamma oscillations increases with greater working memory load (Williams & Boska, 2010). In other words, gamma synchrony increases with the amount of information the working memory holds. This is relevant because patients with schizophrenia commonly demonstrate perturbed working memory (Williams & Boska, 2010). In fact, in a study where healthy subjects and patients with schizophrenia were told to complete a mental arithmetic task, patients with schizophrenia demonstrated reduced gamma activity during the retrieval period of working memory compared to healthy subjects (Haenschel et al., 2009).

Gamma oscillations stimulated by other tasks, not just those that exercise the working memory, also are perturbed in patients with schizophrenia. When patients with chronic and early-onset schizophrenia were exposed to continuous clicking sounds, it was found that gamma oscillations evoked in the auditory cortex had reduced synchrony compared to those in healthy controls (Williams & Boska, 2010). When presented with visual gestalt stimuli (visual stimuli where individual elements form a meaningful whole), patients with schizophrenia showed gamma oscillations of reduced amplitude as well as gamma oscillations of slower frequency (Williams & Boska, 2010). For example, in a study where patients with schizophrenia were presented with images of happy or fearful faces, patients with schizophrenia displayed lower gamma synchrony compared to healthy controls (Williams et al., 2009). Moreover, the reduction in gamma synchrony predicted poorer social cognition (Williams et al., 2009).

The relationship between gamma oscillations and the binding of visual stimuli is an interesting one, because some cognitive scientists believe that synchronous neural firing at the gamma frequency might be the neural correlate of consciousness (Ward, 2003). This is because consciousness is believed to be implied when visual awareness is demonstrated, and visual awareness is demonstrated when visual gestalt stimuli are processed as a meaningful whole (Ward, 2003). The potential relationship between gamma oscillations and consciousness is further demonstrated in an experiment where subjects were shown an ambiguous image which could have been processed as a meaningless shape or a face. When subjects reported seeing a face, gamma synchrony was observed on the EEG recording of subjects, whereas this synchronization was not observed when a meaningless shape was reported (Rodriguez et al., 1999). The connection between gamma synchrony and consciousness has opened larger doors to neuroscientists because it suggests that schizophrenia can be seen as a disorder of consciousness.

When studying a psychiatric disorder, it is always important to consider whether its characteristics may be attributed to medication use. The association between reduced gamma synchrony and schizophrenia is no exception. So far, some research has shown that deficits in neural oscillations are present regardless of medication status, while other research has shown that treatment by certain antipsychotics results in gamma oscillations within the normal range (Uhlhaas & Singer, 2010). Although the research does not fully agree on whether medicated patients with schizophrenia exhibit normal or perturbed neural oscillations, it does agree that non-medicated patients do indeed exhibit abnormal neural oscillations and synchronization at illness onset (Uhlhaas & Singer, 2010). Hence, the observed relationship between gamma synchrony and schizophrenia is not attributable to antipsychotic use.

Theories of Consciousness

Not only has schizophrenia been proposed as being related to consciousness in research on gamma oscillations, but it also has been proposed as a disorder of consciousness in the Orch OR (orchestrated objective reduction) theory. However, before addressing the Orch OR theory and its relationship with schizophrenia, it is worth briefly reviewing the three general theories of consciousness in the universe. The first theory proposes that consciousness is a natural consequence of the evolution of brains and the nervous system, and hence is not an intrinsic feature of the universe (Hameroff & Penrose, 2014). The second theory proposes that consciousness has always been in the universe and lies outside of science, in that it is not controlled by physical laws (Hameroff & Penrose, 2014). Religious and spiritual viewpoints on consciousness, for example, would fall under this umbrella. Finally, the third theory proposes that consciousness arises from discrete (quantum) physical events which have always existed in the universe (Hameroff & Penrose, 2014). This theory suggests that consciousness obeys physical laws, but that biology evolved mechanisms to orchestrate these discrete events and couple them with neuronal activity (Hameroff & Penrose, 2014). This third view is consistent with the Orch OR theory, which posits that consciousness involves quantum processes in the microtubules of neurons (Venkatasubramanian, 2015).

Microtubule Abnormalities in Schizophrenia

Microtubules are cylindrical polymers that are assembled from tubulin proteins (Hameroff & Penrose, 2014). They form the scaffolding of the cell cytoskeleton along with other proteins such as actin (Hameroff & Penrose, 2014). Interestingly, microtubules in neurons have also been proposed to be involved in information processing and computation (Hameroff & Penrose, 2014). This is because microtubules in the dendrites and soma of neurons are uniquely arranged in networks that are suitable for information processing (Hameroff & Penrose, 2014).

The Orch OR theory claims that neuronal microtubule information processing is a result of the quantum processes that occur in the microtubule, ultimately suggesting that this quantum behaviour might underlie the generation of consciousness (Venkatasubramanian, 2015). Unsurprisingly, schizophrenia has also been shown to be associated with microtubule abnormalities (Venkatasubramanian, 2015). One study showed that the distribution of two microtubule-associated proteins (MAPs), MAP2 and MAP5, were significantly altered in five of six patients with schizophrenia (Arnold et al., 1991). Because the arrangement of microtubules is important to cognitive functioning, it is possible that these abnormalities in microtubule arrangement are involved in the pathophysiology of schizophrenia (Arnold et al., 1991). Additionally, another study found that the hyperphosphorylation (saturation of phosphoryl sites) of tau has been associated with schizophrenia (Venkatasubramanian, 2015). Tau is a MAP that regulates microtubule assembly and stability.

Understanding the role of aberrant microtubule arrangement in schizophrenia opens doors to potential treatments for schizophrenia. Certain antipsychotics as well as electroconvulsive therapy involve targeting neuronal microtubules (Venkatasubramanian, 2015). Electroconvulsive therapy is when small electric currents pass through the brain in a patient under general anesthesia to trigger a brief seizure which alters one's brain chemistry.

Criticisms of the Orch OR Theory

The Orch OR theory is controversial and has been criticized ever since it was first proposed. For instance, certain neuroscientists argue that the microtubule-disabling drug colchicine does not cause patients to lose consciousness, and therefore, microtubules cannot be essential for consciousness (Hameroff & Penrose, 2015). In response, supporters of the Orch OR theory noted that colchicine doesn't cross the blood-brain barrier, and thus would not reach neuronal microtubules. Other critics question whether there are enough tubulins for individual quantum processes to result in consciousness (Hameroff & Penrose, 2015).

Conclusion

This chapter reviewed two explanations for the pathophysiology of schizophrenia: aberrant gamma oscillations and microtubule abnormalities. These correspond more generally to the disconnection hypothesis and the Orch OR theory, respectively. What is important to note is that these two hypotheses are not dichotomous; in fact, the Orch OR theory agrees that gamma synchrony is the main measurable indicator of consciousness (Venkatasubramanian, 2015). The Orch OR theory instead explains consciousness, including gamma synchrony, from a quantum biological level. Overall, both theories suggest that schizophrenia can be seen as a disorder of consciousness. This is because aberrant gamma oscillations and microtubule abnormalities, which are proposed to be involved in consciousness, are exhibited in patients with schizophrenia. Moreover, certain symptoms of schizophrenia are consistent with perturbed visual and conscious awareness. Schizophrenia is a complex disorder and is still not completely understood. However, by examining schizophrenia through multiple angles, a more detailed and meaningful picture is painted.

42

CHAPTER 6

The Prodrome and Antecedents of Schizophrenia

Vedanshi Vala

Introduction

"Never surrender, never give up", said Dr. Austin Mardon in sharing his personal motto. From his PhD, to his work with NASA in Antarctica, to his Order of Canada award, and to founding the Antarctic Institute of Canada, Dr. Mardon has to date had an impressive and inspiring career. He has also overcome significant adversity to reach his current position, having experienced discrimination as a person living with schizophrenia.

This chapter will focus on the prodrome and antecedents of schizophrenia, and culminate in a conversation on empathy and inclusion. Schizophrenia is a mental disorder that approximately one percent of people worldwide live with, is chronic, and may be disabling in nature (Insel, 2010). Schizophrenia prodrome "is characterized as a process of changes or deterioration in [...] behavioral symptoms that precede the onset of clinical psychotic symptoms" (Larson et al., 2010, p. 4). On the other hand, the antecedents of schizophrenia refer to the factors which may contribute towards an individual's predisposition to the mental disorder, such as their genetic makeup (Mcglashan and Woods, 2011).

As a person who has lived with schizophrenia for nearly three decades, Dr. Mardon's personal experiences form a significant portion of the contents of this chapter, as shared by him personally in an interview. When asked whether he had personally experienced discrimination due to his mental illness, Dr. Mardon shared how, "as an adult, [he] had many avenues blocked off towards [him]. It's really quite a miracle that [he] was able to" get to where he is today. Just given "the systemic discrimination and the negative things, aside from the limitations of schizophrenia itself, the level of discrimination [he has] encountered" is beyond apprehensible, and is appalling. It is incredibly commendable that Dr. Mardon has overcome such adversity to stand where he is today; however, it is unfortunate and disappointing that he had to experience it in the first place. This serves as a reminder on the need to actively combat stigma, and flip such oppressive narratives. As such, the objective of this chapter is to highlight the disparities experienced by people living with mental illness, in an effort to break the stigma, and build the current narrative into a more inclusive one.

Schizophrenia Prodrome: Signs and Symptoms

As mentioned in the introduction, schizophrenia prodrome is the phase which precedes, and may escalate into, the clinical psychosis stage. Notably, those who experience "poor functioning, long duration of symptoms, high levels of depression, reduced attention and family history and deterioration of functioning paired with experiencing subthreshold psychotic symptoms" are more likely to move out of the prodromal phase of schizophrenia and experience clinical psychosis (Larson et al., 2010, p. 5). However, this also means that treating symptoms experienced in the prodrome can potentially prevent the illness from developing into psychosis (Insel, 2010).

Speaking from his own experience, Dr. Mardon shared some of the symptoms he experienced in the prodromal phase. "I couldn't read body language", he said, "and I had mistrust, depression, anxiety, social isolation—those were major ones." Due to the loss of focus he experienced, as a strategy for coping, Dr. Mardon tried to just "stick to one thing" because he "didn't really want to flip back and forth between things". This was prior to his official diagnosis between the years of 1991 and 1992; however, Dr. Mardon's childhood doctors said that he had schizophrenia back in 1985. In explaining this discrepancy, Dr. Mardon said that, "there were seven years between, probably, when I developed it and when I was actually diagnosed—which is not that uncommon. A lot of people go on for years of dysfunction before they get put on meds—or properly put on meds." Such a period is classified as 'untreated psychosis', which can last from several weeks to many years—as in Dr. Mardon's case (Mcglashan and Woods, 2011). This can certainly raise questions about whether better education about symptoms of the prodromal phase is needed. However, Dr. Mardon shared a different perspective.

"Well, the problem is a lot more people are prodromal in the gene pool than actually develop schizophrenia. So a lot of people will have those issues that will never develop schizophrenia." As such, as Dr. Mardon continued to explain, there are limitations to what can be done in the prodromal phase, aside from individuals who are genetically predisposed to schizophrenia taking folic acid, fish oil, and talk therapy. Dr. Mardon then spoke about the onset of prodromal symptoms in teenagers. "The number of kids that have those characteristics, it's—a lot of adolescents have depression, not all of them develop schizophrenia." Given this, Dr. Mardon established how talk therapy earlier would be beneficial "for the whole population long-term—people would be getting more stabilized". However, "you wouldn't want to medicate adolescents" because in the developing age, "that would affect their brains".

Ultimately, to echo what Dr. Mardon said, while having certain symptoms in the prodromal phase or genetic history can make someone more predisposed to schizophrenia, those indicators alone do not guarantee the development of psychosis. As a result, implementing earlier identifiers for the prodromes of schizophrenia and coping strategies, such as talk therapy, may be an effective strategy to better health outcomes. The next section in this chapter will focus on the treatment of this illness, and its antecedents.

Antecedents of Schizophrenia: Diagnosis and Treatment

The antecedents of schizophrenia are the variables determining predisposition to the illness, as discussed in the introduction. For one, individuals with a family history of schizophrenia must be considered for genetic vulnerability to the illness (Mcglashan and Woods, 2011). Moreover, nuances in childhood and adolescent development may also have an impact on the development of schizophrenia in adulthood (Welham et al., 2008). When evaluated for the purposes of a diagnosis, the DSM-5 definition of psychosis is used as a guideline; however, it should be noted that until an individual meets the threshold for such a diagnosis, the symptoms would be classified as either 'prodromal' or 'psychosis-risk' (Mcglashan and Woods, 2011). There is considerable debate in psychiatry over whether the psychosis-risk symptoms should be an entirely new DSM-5 classification as a syndrome, which would recognize the prodromal phase of schizophrenia as "a legitimate, and important, clinical entity" of its own (Mcglashan and Woods, 2011, para. 20).

After an individual exhibits prodromal symptoms, there are several factors which psychologists must consider in developing treatment plans for their patients, given the presence of both risks and benefits to earlier intervention (Mcglashan and Woods, 2011). For one, there is debate over whether patients who are in the prodromal phase of the illness should be prescribed medication, or whether their symptoms should be monitored until they can be classified as schizophrenic (Mcglashan and Woods, 2011). Medication can have side effects, such as the drug olanzapine causing weight gain, which needs to be evaluated against the ability to treat prodromal symptoms before they escalate into clinical psychosis (Mcglashan and Woods, 2011).

In response to a question about challenges he had experienced with the use of medication as part of his treatment plan, Dr. Mardon answered that "it's very difficult to be so disciplined". His treatment plan requires taking medication "every day, twice a day for what has been now almost 29 years". When asked how he maintained such a difficult routine, Dr. Mardon pointed to the quote he'd shared earlier from the Galaxy Quest movie, "never surrender, never give up". Despite his mental strength, there were some taxing physical hardships Dr.

Mardon had to combat while taking his medication. "Originally, the medication was quite toxic. You know, it's like I was a zombie. But in '96 I changed to the atypical neuroleptic class of medication that started with risperidone- and I started getting more cognition back". The process of switching from the first type of medication he took to the risperidone, which was much better suited to him, required Dr. Mardon to have in-depth conversations with his medical team. This included discussion on how his previous medication affected him and his body personally, and then navigating towards the better option afterwards. "But, I mean I just had to take it." Dr. Mardon had observed his mother, who wasn't as cooperative with taking the medication required of her own treatment plan, and having witnessed the outcome, he "didn't want to repeat that." As a result, Dr. Mardon attributes his motivation to that incident. "A lot of the reasoning, I think, in my head was internal fear."

If an individual is struggling with taking medication regularly, Dr. Mardon asserted that it is not discriminatory to tell them to follow their treatment plan—it is important that they be, in fact, encouraged and supported throughout their treatment. However, Dr. Mardon emphasized that "there are a lot of side effects. So if somebody's doing that, they're doing their best. They're doing, probably, more in their lives than anybody else is doing. They're sacrificing a lot." Side effects can deter an individual from taking their medication, such as "the diabetes, the thyroid damage, the obesity [...]. Like, if somebody's doing all this stuff, then it's quite difficult. I mean, I don't think most people would take the meds that would cause diabetes and impotence. [...] Yet every male who takes schizophrenia meds is doing that. You know, that really affects people. So they should be encouraged to stay on their meds and given a fair shot. [...] They don't need to be discriminated [against] so much" simply because they are a person with a disability or mental illness.

Beyond medication, there are other aspects to Dr. Mardon's personal treatment and management plan for schizophrenia. For one, "finding a purpose. The blue zone, which is talking about concentrations of where centaurians are in the world" looks at people who live long lives, "they attribute it to something called a 'khagi', which [means] 'your purpose in life'. And I felt that the purpose in my life was the writing, and the students, my foster sons, and my relationship with Catherine." In discussing factors which are stressors to his symptoms, Dr. Mardon said, "Well, when our foster sons aren't doing well, or the fact that I have to loan 80 thousand dollars every year [...] that's a great financial pressure every year." This highlights how socioeconomic factors can exacerbate the vulnerabilities of those living with a mental illness, and as such, minimizing the impact of such pressures may promote improved mental health.

Dr. Mardon's family forms his support network, and they work together to support him in the process of treating and managing schizophrenia. Beyond his family, there are many ways in which individuals in the community can foster a safer space for Dr. Mardon and other people living with mental illness. The next section explores this very topic.

Breaking the Stigma: Empathy and Inclusion

Through increased understanding about schizophrenia's prodromal symptoms, its antecedents and treatments, society can strive towards improved inclusion for people living with the mental illness. Empathy, understanding, and respect are at the foundation of fostering a more inclusive society.

Dr. Mardon shared his own experiences being bullied in childhood as the son of a parent who had schizophrenia. "I experienced discrimination as a child before I developed schizophrenia, because my mother had schizophrenia, from the other kids and the other people in our neighbourhood." A particular study examining the discrimination experienced by people with schizophrenia and their relatives resounds with Dr. Mardon's experiences (González-Torres et al., 2006). In the study, the researchers examined discrimination in several instances, such as over-protection and infantilization, in daily social activities, in health care, by children of parents with mental illness, and social isolation, as experienced by both patients and their relatives (González-Torres et al., 2006). The study concluded that both patients and relatives encountered stigma and discrimination, and to escape such a reality, many people resorted to isolation (González-Torres et al., 2006). Recognizing that such discrimination is present in society is one of the first steps towards eradicating it down the road, so that patients with schizophrenia have better health outcomes (González-Torres et al., 2006).

In addressing how, as a person living with schizophrenia, he feels people can be more inclusive and supportive of him and other people with mental illness, Dr. Mardon emphasized increased compassion and lack of prejudice. "Take me for who I am. You might not like me for what I am, but just give me a fair choice and fair chance, and don't discriminate against me. Don't think I'm a monster, because—as I say—you shouldn't be afraid of me, you should be afraid of my wife, 'cuz she's a lawyer."

When asked whether Dr. Mardon felt at any point that he was seen differently when people learned that he lives with schizophrenia, he shared an anecdote from the day he received his Order of Canada and conversed with the Governor General of Canada at the time, Michelle Jean, in Rideau Hall. "I was standing in the middle of the room. Michelle Jean and her entourage were working their way over, and eventually she [came] over and [my wife] Catherine was standing about ten feet away. Then, Michelle Jean [started] talking and she touched my shoulder and we had a very in-depth conversation about mental illness—she's done stuff with mental illness in her career." Meanwhile, "Catherine was observing what was actually happening around me and Michelle Jean, and what happened was her security team [...] was surrounding her. What happened was, they put their hands on their jackets, and they were looking like they weren't blinking, and they were looking like they were ready to pounce, because a schizophrenic was talking to [the Governor General]. And when she reached out to touch me, they almost had a seizure—they were just standing there, ready to jump. And then, on and on it goes. [...] You have to understand that everybody in that audience was either family members or members of the Order of Canada, or members of the Supreme Court—they were all vetted. And most of them were, and I was vetted too. So even if my most senior, highest honour I have was the Order of Canada—they were still deathly afraid of me. You know, like I was more terrified than the Governor General, afraid I'd trip or throw up or something. And so, they were even afraid of me. So disappointing."

Given that misinterpretation of body language is a prodrome of schizophrenia that Dr. Mardon personally experiences, he noted that this event was observed and interpreted by his wife, Catherine. He continued his anecdote, sharing how "as soon as [the Governor General] moved away, [her security detail] all relaxed, and were talking to each other." Dr. Mardon continued to say that with the Order of Canada being "my greatest honour, my family's greatest honour, [in this] generation... And they're still afraid of me." This incident in particular made Dr. Mardon feel that "there's no way [...] discrimination is gonna change. So I wanted to just forget about it." This incident is difficult to digest, but is demonstrative of the stigma embedded in society against people with mental illness. "Why did they give me an award if they were afraid of me?" was what Dr. Mardon asked.

Dr. Mardon's experiences are unfortunately unsurprising, given that people who live with mental illness are more likely to be subjected to violence than they are to physically attack others (Stuart, 2003). Violence comes from a place of socioeconomic disparities and substance abuse, and while these factors may coincide with mental illness, it is not the stem of violence itself (Stuart, 2003). That people with mental illness are a threat to others is a misconception, and Dr. Mardon's experiences reiterate how their alienation from society is a direct result of this discrimination. Rectifying underlying issues of financial stress, aiming for earlier identification of drug or alcohol dependency, and providing management strategies for substance abuse disorders can curb the cause of violence from its root (Stuart, 2003).

In reflecting upon a sweet and considerate moment where another individual's actions helped him cope with schizophrenia, Dr. Mardon remarked that "When I met the Pope, the Pope didn't punch me for kissing his ring [...] and he didn't just leave, he kept talking to us." Given how much this event meant to him, even though it seems as simple as another person taking the time to have a conversation, it highlights the importance of seeing people for who they truly are; their mental illness shouldn't be used to define who they are as a person.

When asked what he would like to remind readers of, Dr. Mardon shared how there are many "horror stories" about the difficulties of coping with mental illness, "but compared to the past" when his great-grandmother and mother battled mental illness, "life has hope today" due to improvements in the medication used in treatment. "And yet, a lot of people don't avail themselves of it because of systemic discrimination. People observing that, and not wanting to have a label or any admission of guilt of being sick" do not take the medication they need to manage their illness. This statement in particular demonstrates how discrimination hinders those who require support and treatment from accessing it. "You know, it's [not] surprising then, there's so much discrimination against people with schizophrenia, and people are willing to do anything to not admit they have it."

As highlighted by what was said by Dr. Mardon, discrimination first affects people who have come forward to say that they have a disability or mental illness, and that they are doing their best to treat it, to cope with it, and to live with it. Then there are people who are afraid to step up to do so because they have witnessed the extent of the discrimination, thereby avoiding the support they need to treat and manage their illness. Ultimately, re-education, change in mentality, and re-writing the discriminatory narrative is incredibly important for creating an inclusive community for people living with mental illness. It is attributed to leaders like Dr. Mardon, who advocate for the rights of those with mental illness, that society can learn and progress in a better direction.

Conclusion

This chapter focused on the prodrome and antecedents of schizophrenia, with an emphasis on empathy and inclusion for people living with the mental illness. In a personal interview, Dr. Austin Mardon shared the grim reality about the adversity he experienced as a person living with schizophrenia, which was complemented by findings in literature. Individuals with mental illness shouldn't have to put themselves on a pedestal and fight for respect, for dignity, and for the world to recognize them as fellow human beings.

"Don't think I'm a monster."

CHAPTER 7

Treatments for Schizophrenia

Sara Djeddi

Introduction

Schizophrenia is a severe and chronic mental illness which is accompanied by various symptoms affecting cognition and behaviour (Patel et al., 2014). These symptoms include "delusions, hallucinations, disorganized speech or behavior, and impaired cognitive ability", giving these patients an altered sense of reality (Patel et al., 2014). Schizophrenia is a difficult illness to bear for both individuals affected and their families (Patel et al., 2014). The illness is often referred to as disabling because of its accompanying symptoms (Patel et al., 2014). Specifically, its negative symptoms, which are associated with a loss or deficit of function such as lack of speech, and its cognitive symptoms, for instance attention impairment (Patel et al., 2014). Positive symptoms of schizophrenia, which are additions to normal functioning, such as hallucinations and delusions, are a possible cause of relapses (Patel et al., 2014). In general, the aim of schizophrenia treatment is to relieve symptoms, prevent relapse, as well as prepare patients for societal integration via their behaviour (Patel et al., 2014).

Psychotherapies

In the case of psychosocial treatments, it is important to understand that the illness goes beyond its immediate medical symptoms (Patel et al., 2014). Schizophrenia takes a toll on the individuals themselves, including "isolation from families and friends; damage to social and working relationships; depression and demoralization; and an increased risk of self-harm, aggression, and substance abuse" (Addington et al., 2010, p. 260). Psychosocial treatment, focusing on society, for schizophrenia is crucial which is why most treatment guidelines include it alongside psychological methods (Addington et al., 2010). In addition to therapy centered around the individual, other programs that focus on patients' families are promising in decreasing rehospitalization and increasing socialization (Patel et al., 2014). These programs are involved in most psychotherapies and target social support where family members learn to look out for the patient (Patel et al., 2014). The chances of patients returning to their previous adaptive functioning are low, which is why both pharmacological and psychosocial approaches are needed for optimal long-term improvement (Patel et al., 2014). Drug therapy is very common with treating schizophrenia though it leaves residual symptoms (Patel et al., 2014). Interestingly, non-pharmacological treatments, such as psychosocial treatments, have been proven to be useful in reducing some of these left over symptoms (Patel et al., 2014).

Psychotherapies are branched into three different categories: individual, group, and cognitive behavioral; these treatment categories are continuously evolving (Patel et al., 2014). It is important to understand that this form of treatment should not be used as a replacement for pharmacological ones, rather they should be implemented as an addition (Patel et al., 2014). Meta-cognitive training, narrative therapies, and mindfulness therapy are examples of common psychotherapies (Patel et al., 2014). For instance, mindfulness therapy focuses on meditation, which in turn can decrease symptoms of schizophrenia (Patel et al., 2014). In addition to being useful in reducing symptomes, psychotherapies can be used to ensure that patients with schizophrenia adhere to their pharmacological treatments (Patel et al., 2014). Those with mental disorders have a tendency to not be very adherent to their medication schedules, specifically, the rate of nonadherence ranges from 37% to 74% for patients with schizophrenia (Patel et al., 2014). This is because "they may deny their illness; they may experience adverse effects that dissuade them from taking more medication; they may not perceive their need for medication; or they may have grandiose symptoms or paranoia" (Patel et al., 2014, p. 641). When a patient stops their pharmacological treatment, it increases the likelihood of their relapse and hospitalization (Patel et al., 2014). Consequently, it is crucial that patients with schizophrenia consistently take their medication and that they become educated about their illness and its respective treatments (Patel et al., 2014). For instance, cognitive behavioral therapy (CBT), personal therapy, and compliance therapy are all examples of psychotherapies that are able to explain the importance of the adherence of medication to patients with schizophrenia (Patel et al., 2014).

Cognitive behavioral therapy (CBT) is generally used as a treatment method for anxiety and depression, but has more recently been shown to be effective for schizophrenia (Addington et al., 2010). Specifically, it is used to treat patients' first psychosis episodes, where they lose their sense of reality (Addington et al., 2010). CBT is a "hierarchical patient-oriented approach to treatment that draws on a diverse array of texts and treatment protocols using empirically supported intervention strategies that have been written up as manuals" (Addington et al., 2010, p. 261). Individuals with schizophrenia are known to have delusions which differ qualitatively, meaning in nature, from processes that are non-delusional (Addington et al., 2010). However, specific features of these delusions, such as conviction (how convinced the patient is that their delusions are real), significance, intensity, and inflexibility, are common in psychotic and non-psychotic conditions (Addington et al., 2010). CBT works by focusing on these listed features, and follows the premise that patients' behaviour is a result of biological factors such as genetics (Addington et al., 2010). Moreover, this treatment addresses engagement, education, adaptation, comorbid anxiety and depression, coping strategies, relapse prevention, and reduction of positive and negative symptoms (Addington et al., 2010). Research has demonstrated the addition of CBT along with pharmacotherapy can "improve symptoms, reduce relapse, and potentially enhance functional capacity and overall life quality" (Addington et al., 2010, p. 261).

Pharmacological Treatments

Beginning pharmacological treatment promptly is crucial, this is due to the fact that the brain of patients with schizophrenia experiences its most extensive changes during the first five years of the illness (Patel et al., 2014). For the majority of these patients, antipsychotic agents, also known as neuroleptic drugs, are needed in order to see progress in their rehabilitation as these drugs with psychotic episodes (Patel et al., 2014). Furthermore, it is also important that these agents are given to patients immediately if they are experiencing an acute episode (Patel et al., 2014). The first seven days of drug therapy are critical, as they will determine the suitable dosage for said patient (Patel et al., 2014). This first week focuses on decreasing the patients hostility, in order to get their functionality back to the standard (Patel et al., 2014). Once the acute phase with pharmacological treatment has passed, the new goal with maintenance therapy is to improve the patients' mood, self-care, and socialization, as well as to prevent relapse (Patel et al., 2014). Patients with schizophrenia that have received maintenance therapy have a rate of relapse of 18 to 32% as compared to 60 to 80% in those without maintenance treatment (Patel et al., 2014). Therapy using neuroleptic drugs should persist for a minimum of one year after a patient's first psychotic episode (Patel et al., 2014). If a change in antipsychotic is needed, before doing so, the medical history of the patient is required in order to use previous response to prior treatments as a guide (Patel et al., 2014).

The American Psychiatric Association has stated that second-generation antipsychotics (SGAs), other than clozapine, are the main drugs used for the initial treatment of schizophrenia (Patel et al., 2014). The two types of antipsychotics are SGAs and first-generation (typical) antipsychotics, FGAs (Patel et al., 2014). SGAs have an impact on patients' metabolic systems, causing weight gain, hyperlipidemia (high cholesterol), and diabetes mellitus (Patel et al., 2014). Nonetheless, they are still favoured over FGAs, as the latter has a greater amount of adverse side effects and symptoms (Patel et al., 2014). The SGA clozapine is of concern due to the threat of agranulocytosis, a severe condition where the body does not produce enough neutrophils (white blood cells) resulting in a suppressed immune system (Patel et al., 2014). Although it is not readily recommended, clozapine has been shown to be effective specifically for patients with schizophrenia under the age of 35 and has been shown to decrease the risk of suicide to a greater degree than other neuroleptics such as olanzapine (Vanesse et al., 2016). Despite the higher chance of hospitalization and death, it has also been shown to decrease the likelihood of physical health events (Vanesse et al., 2016). In addition to this, clozapine, quetiapine, olanzapine and risperidone all decrease patients' risk of stopping or changing drugs when compared to FGAs (Vanesse et al., 2016).

A pharmacotherapeutic algorithm has been suggested by The Texas Medication Algorithm Project (TMAP) in order to treat patients with schizophrenia (Patel et al., 2014). The first stage following this algorithm consists of treatment with a single SGA (Patel et al., 2014). The following step, stage 2, begins if the patient has no response or little response to that SGA and continues with monotherapy of a different SGA or in some cases an FGA (Patel et al., 2014). If the patient also has no response to stage 2, stage 3 can begin, where the patient begins a course of clozapine while their white blood cell (WBC) count is monitored to the risk of agranulocytosis (Patel et al., 2014). If agranulocytosis occurs, the use of clozapine will be halted (Patel et al., 2014). Once again, with little to no response comes the following step: stage 4 (Patel et al., 2014). In this stage, treatment consists of a combination of clozapine with either an FGA, an SGA, or electroconvulsive therapy (ECT) (Patel et al., 2014). Next, stage 5 is similar to stage 2, where a single FGA or SGA that has yet to be used is administered for therapy (Patel et al., 2014). If stage 5 does not produce results, the last phase, stage 6, can begin, which is combination therapy of an SGA, an FGA, ECT, or a mood stabilizer (Patel et al., 2014). As mentioned, combining drugs should only be attempted at the end of the algorithm because taking multiple antipsychotic agents can increase the risk of drug interactions, nonadherence, and medication errors (Patel et al., 2014).

Treatment Resistance

Patients with schizophrenia that are treatment-resistant can be defined as those who "despite at least two adequate trials of classical neuroleptic drugs, have persistent moderate to severe positive, or disorganisation, or negative symptoms together with poor social and work function over a prolonged period of time" (Meltzer, 1997, p. 1). Using this definition, 10 to 45% of individuals with schizophrenia are considered resistant to treatment (Meltzer, 1997). Moreover, approximately 30 to 60% of patients with schizophrenia have adverse side effects as well as minimal improvement as a result of antipsychotic treatments (Patel et al., 2014). Due to their symptoms and behaviour, treatment-resistant patients with schizophrenia are prone to more hospitalizations with longer visits, resulting in care and treatment that are significantly more expensive (Meltzer, 1997). Despite their early treatment resistance, a portion of these individuals will spontaneously begin to respond to treatments or start to develop less symptoms (Meltzer, 1997).

Treatment-resistant patients with schizophrenia begin to develop positive symptoms earlier, and are often male (Meltzer, 1997). In addition, they have inferior premorbid function as well as ventricular abnormalities, which was discovered using computer and imagining technologies (Meltzer, 1997). In other words, these patients suffer from lower cognitive function prior to having schizophrenia, as well as abnormal heartbeats (Meltzer, 1997). When comparing individuals with schizophrenia and those with treatment-resistant schizophrenia, a difference is seen in cognitive impairment, which is more acute (more severe) in the latter (Meltzer, 1997).

Patients with treatment-resistant schizophrenia do not typically exhibit a response to an increase in dosage or a change in their current antipsychotic drug (Meltzer, 1997). Additionally, secondary drugs and agents such as benzodiazepines, antidepressants, anticonvulsants, and lithium carbonate have no effect on these individuals (Meltzer, 1997). However, the aforementioned drug clozapine, appears to be the most effective in the management of patients with treatment-resistant schizophrenia (Patel et al., 2014). The problem with clozapine lies with the safety of its use (Patel et al., 2014). This antipsychotic drug can increase patients' risks at developing orthostatic hypotension, a type of low blood pressure, and can cause severe consequences if taken at high doses (Patel et al., 2014). Despite its risks, clozapine is more promising than the majority of other antipsychotic drugs in "decreasing psychopathology, improving some aspects of cognition, improving quality of life, decreasing hospitalisation, and decreasing suicide attempts and completions" (Meltzer, 1997, p. 3). Of those with treatment-resistant schizophrenia that take clozapine, 20% experience almost no positive symptoms and 40% are capable of finishing school or working (Meltzer, 1997). This drug is also useful in managing the blood sodium levels for individuals with low concentrations of sodium or those with extreme thirstiness (Patel et al., 2014).

Conclusion

The treatment of patients with schizophrenia is crucial, especially following their first psychotic episode (Patel et al., 2014). It is also important to consider treatment-resistance patients with schizophrenia, as there are a variety of methods available to aid them. Although both psychotherapies and pharmacological treatments are useful in increasing adaptive functioning in patients with schizophrenia, further research should focus on curing this chronic mental illness (Patel et al., 2014).

CHAPTER 8

The Effects of Being a Spouse of a Person with Schizophrenia

Lilian Yeung

Introduction

Mental health is an important aspect of wellbeing besides physical health. Within the realm of mental health includes the various mental illnesses or disorders that a person may have. A significant mental health disorder is schizophrenia; a long-term neurodevelopmental disorder which is characterized by mental fragmentation where a person may suffer from psychotic symptoms such as delusions and disorganization (Kahn et al., 2015). Schizophrenia is an exceptionally complex syndrome as it is a psychiatric disorder that can be triggered by both environmental factors and genetics (Jungbauer et al., 2004). Because schizophrenia manifests differently in each individual, along with the onset of illness being hard to identify, the treatment of schizophrenia will also vary though it will typically include both medication and psychological therapy (Jungbauer et al., 2004). In addition, schizophrenia has no cure and treatments made are to improve one's quality of life by reducing the symptoms and also helping to prevent future symptoms (C. Mardon, personal communication, August 5, 2021). Even though much research has been conducted on schizophrenia and there have been many improvements on the treatment and quality of life for those affected by schizophrenia, there still remains much unknown in this mental disorder and more improvements needed.

Due to the timeline of schizophrenia's onset, which may begin during early adolescent years, it can severely impact a person's developing mind along with their social and cognitive skills, which are critical in becoming an independently functional social being (Kahn et al., 2015). Although these skills will start to decline, they are often not perceived as the onset of schizophrenia until psychotic symptoms start to appear which may take more than 10 years afterwards (Kahn et al., 2015). With the onset and schizophrenia effects varying for each individual, patients' recovery may range from a chronic need of management to a complete recovery, although most individuals with this disorder will still have a reduced lifespan—by 20 years—as compared to the general population (Kahn et al., 2015). A complete recovery does not mean that the person has been cured of schizophrenia, but rather has sufficient management of symptoms related to schizophrenia and thus is able to live a life relatively unaffected by schizophrenia (Kahn et al., 2015). Schizophrenia affects all aspects of life, especially the ability to retain employment, build and maintain social relationships, and live independently (Kahn et al., 2015). Thus, those who are severely impacted by schizophrenia may need a caregiver and a support network to help improve their quality of life and regain independence in their daily life.

Support for People Living with Schizophrenia

Oftentimes, this support network comes in the form of family and friends. The care that family provides is invaluable to a person with chronic mental illness, but it can also take a toll on the family members themselves. This toll has been termed as 'burden of care' (Kumari et al., 2009). Burden of care is a complex term that has no simple definitions but rather encapsulates and is defined by the impacts and effects caregivers experience when caring for those with a chronic illness (Kumari et al., 2009). Such impacts include emotional, physical, psychological and economic impact (Kumari et al., 2009). When the term 'burden of care' was first conceptualized, there were 2 classifications in which there was subjective and objective burden of care (Kumari et al., 2009). The subjective burden of care includes the emotional and psychological effects of mental illness such as feelings of sorrow and anxiety while the objective burden of care includes the physical effects on the family—for example, taking care of chores or physical tasks (Kumari et al., 2009). The care provided by a spouse of schizophrenia is a long lasting stressor and comes with a substantial amount of burden (Kumari et al., 2009). It not only affects the spouse but also the rest of the family. In cases where a person is affected with a severe form of schizophrenia, their family experiences a greater overall burden to care for them (Kumari et al., 2009).

Furthermore, there is much stigma that continues to shadow mental illness in current society. Although there have been many advances in removing the stigma and fear of mental illness, the majority of the public still lacks awareness and understanding of mental disorders (Jungbauer et al., 2004). The media also continues to perpetuate much of the stereotypes and stigma attached to schizophrenia, and does not show the full scope of what this mental disorder encompasses. In spite of the fact that improvements have been made to bring awareness and understanding to mental disorders, people still fear those with mental illness and ostracise them (Kelly, 2005). Society tends to immediately latch onto a person's mental disorder and treat it as the whole identity of the person or using it as a derogatory word (Kelly, 2005). Hence, most people do not take the time to separate the person themselves from their mental illness or disorders as shown with the terms 'schizophrenic', 'retard', etc when featured in movies such as Tropic Thunder. These terms all have negative connotations and are often used in derogatory ways. So the continued use of such terms in media and literary works will only add to the struggle that those with mental illness face when interacting with society and asserting their independence.

Catherine Mardon, a Canadian lawyer and activist who has raised awareness of mental disorders and illness, has mentioned that people need to look beyond a person's mental illness to view them as a person (C. Mardon, personal communication, August 5, 2021). She stated that "it is very easy to want to infantilize a mentally ill person" because they may need additional aid in their daily lives, but that we need to acknowledge their capabilities and know that their struggles do not define them.

Spouse of a Person Living with Schizophrenia

As a spouse of Austin Mardon, who is an advocate for mental health along with being a professor and presiding on many councils in addition to having schizophrenia, Catherine Mardon has a unique perspective on what being a spouse of someone with schizophrenia is like. In her situation, she met Austin Mardon, her husband, when he had lived for some time with his mental illness. Within the first few weeks of dating, Austin was upfront about his mental illness of having schizophrenia and revealed the full scope of it to her (C. Mardon, personal communication, August 5, 2021). Since she had experiences interacting with people who have mental disorders through her work along with a deep understanding of what a person who has schizophrenia experiences, her initial reaction to his diagnosis was not one of fear or revulsion, but of understanding, acceptance, and the willingness to look beyond his mental illness to get to know the person he is (C. Mardon, personal communication, August 5, 2021). Most people who are ignorant about mental illnesses are not willing to enter a relationship with someone who has it. Their knowledge of schizophrenia will most likely come from the media and how schizophrenia is portrayed there, which is generally that they are a danger and will hurt people around them. In Catherine's case, she was informed by Austin that he was taking his medications regularly as he was extremely upfront and open about his illness (C. Mardon, personal communication, August 5, 2021). Having open conversations and trust is key in any long lasting stable relationship.

Not only does Catherine understand how schizophrenia affects a person, but she is also able to empathize with that person because of her own trauma and shared experiences. She herself has also suffered an inability to trust her senses, similar to how those with schizophrenia may lose ability to to trust their perceptions (C. Mardon, personal communication, August 5, 2021). Her relationship with Austin has been a positive and supportive stable relationship where they both mutually benefit from this relationship. In many cases, individuals with schizophrenia will generally be unable to live in stable partnerships due to the somewhat early onset of schizophrenia and its illness-related consequences (Kumari et al., 2009). Spouses of people with schizophrenia have to endure schizophrenia-related burdens in addition to burdens that relationships and family roles have (Jungbauer et al., 2004). Thus, spouses of people with schizophrenia must have evaluated their relationship with that person and decided that their partnership gives sufficient support, love, trust, and safety to them in spite of the additional burdens that they may face. The spouses must decide that their quality of life is enriched through this partnership and that they derive happiness from it, hence why they decide to pursue this relationship (Jungbauer et al., 2004). Although relationships or partnerships with people who have schizophrenia can be at risk of disintegration and separation, they are quite often maintained for a number of years (Jungbauer et al., 2004). Long-lasting partnerships appear to be the result of the partner's schizophrenia impairment being perceived as moderate and that the frequency of psychotic episodes occurring is limited and viewed as tolerable to the partner (Jungbauer et al., 2004). Typically, in stable long lasting relationships involving a spouse who has a mental illness, oftentimes their partner may also have mental illness or disabilities themselves, and as such, often encounter this relationship with each other as an acceptable and suitable lifestyle (Jungbauer et al., 2004). This provides additional support for Catherine's relationship with Austin and part of the reason behind them having a long stable relationship with one another. Furthermore, there is mutual understanding and shared experiences that allows spouses to relate to one another more easily and experience more in common which in turn helps strengthen their relationships (Jungbauer et al., 2004).

Research into Spouses of Schizophrenia

There has been a lack of research in the past within the field of spouses of people with schizophrenia which could be explained by the lack of selection when researchers are recruiting study participants (Kumari et al., 2009). Due to economic and practicality, study participants are typically garnered from the pool of self-help groups and caregiver associations, which are mainly parents (Kumari et al., 2009). Additionally, not many people with schizophrenia have a spouse or romantic partner due to misinformation, fear and stigma associated with mental illness in current society (Kelly, 2005). Besides these reasons, most people do not want to take on extra burdens of caring for someone with schizophrenia.

According to Kumari et al. (2009) and other studies, it seems that females with schizophrenia tend to have increased chances of having a spouse or stable partnership than their male counterparts. The 2008 study conducted by Kumari et al. (2009) explored 50 married subjects (25 male and 25 female patients with schizophrenia); they report that different degrees of burden are experienced by spouses of both genders of people with schizophrenia. This indicates that the degree of burden is particular to gender (Kumari et al., 2009). Moreover, their study suggests that considerable mental illnesses or disorders will in due course lead to a perceived subjective burden imposed on the spouse in addition to interrupted interpersonal relationships (Kumari et al., 2009). Lastly, their study concluded that 96% of spouses of females with schizophrenia were employed as opposed to only 28% of spouses of males with schizophrenia were employed (Kumari et al., 2009). Regardless of gender though, both male and female spouses reported experiencing a moderate amount of burden as an outcome of their partner's schizophrenia (Kumari et al., 2009). Jungbauer and colleagues (2004) also reasoned that little research was conducted into spouses of schizophrenia since families and parental relationships remain the most long-term vital exposure to social contact for most people living with schizophrenia.

Also, it has been suggested in numerous studies that patients with a comparatively favourable or moderate course of schizophrenia have increased chances of finding a spouse and maintaining their partnership (Jungbauer et al., 2004). Relationships, especially close relationships or partnerships such as ones of a romantic nature, play an important role in ameliorating the prognosis of schizophrenia for the patient by providing a necessary protective factor (Jungbauer et al., 2004). Like in any relationship, individuals benefit from having a person to confide in and to lean on for support, irrespective of whether they have a mental illness or not. Relationships where one or more partners have a mental illness reinforces the need for someone to trust in and support them. But spouses of a person with mental illness need to also take care of themselves and their mental health before they have the capacity and support needed to enter into a partnership with someone who has a mental illness. During an interview with Catherine, she stresses that "it is not the fact that someone has a disability, it is how you adapt to it and accept it which makes all the difference to whether you are happy or not" (C. Mardon, personal communication, August 5, 2021). Catherine's acceptance of Austin's mental illness and their relationship stems from her own acceptance of herself, as she is physically disabled, and understanding the limitations and benefits within this relationship (C. Mardon, personal communication, August 5, 2021).

The sudden onset of schizophrenia within a couple is a significantly difficult time and can cause extreme burdens on the spouse due to initial psychotic symptoms happening while the spouse of the person affected is unknowledgeable or powerless to help (Jungbauer et al., 2004). Initial psychotic episodes may also be dismissed and not classified (as a symptom or indicator) at all since the behaviour and symptoms of the spouse may be irrational and inexplicable, in addition to a lack of support information available (Jungbauer et al., 2004). Moreover, this situation can evoke feelings of helplessness, fear, worry and despair (Jungbauer et al., 2004).

Partnerships in which the onset of illness has already occured for a patient means that the spouse of the person affected may have a 'sense' or 'theory' of possible risks and burdens with living with a person with schizophrenia (Jungbauer et al., 2004). Spouses of individuals affected may not have a complete picture of all the risks connected to an acute symptom of the illness in addition to also not correctly anticipating the burdens related with schizophrenia (Jungbauer et al., 2004). Ultimately, the more prepared a spouse is in terms of understanding schizophrenia, and what to expect from their partner's illness will help in having a stable and long lasting relationship. Moreover, a spouse able to be knowledgeable about their partner's triggers may help to prevent future symptoms and also reduce the stressors related to schizophrenia.

Catherine Mardon's 3 Important Recommendations for Spouses or Caregivers of a Person with Schizophrenia

Firstly, Catherine stresses the importance of separating the person from the illness (C. Mardon, personal communication, August 5, 2021). When interacting with someone who has a mental illness, it also entails potentially experiencing their symptoms of such mental illness. Therefore, it is key that a spouse or caregiver does not get mad at the person with their mental disorders but rather at the symptoms and illness itself. She also explains how as a spouse of someone with schizophrenia, she does not try to infantilize him, but treats him as a wife would (such as making fun of him and not treating him as a nurse would). Also, in situations where Austin may experience paranoia due to being overstressed and tired, Catherine explains that she would not play into his fears or undermine his thoughts or feelings, but instead acknowledge his feelings and add in her own suggestion to effectively stop his train of thought. This could include telling him that he should hang up the phone if he feels paranoia of someone listening in to his conversations. This method works by not elevating his fears and seeks to deescalate the situation through redirection of one's thoughts and actions.

The second recommendation is to take care of oneself first before taking care of others. Self-care is needed to help a spouse or caregiver to destress, unwind, and look after their own mental health. Self-care may also be different and vary for each person depending on their preferences and experiences. If personal mental health is not first taken care of, a spouse or caregiver will be sacrificing their own mental health to help others, which is harmful to both patients and the caregiver as they are not receiving and giving the best that they could. Catherine mentioned that she enjoys sewing, playing the trombone, and going to visit the cadets as her form of self-care (C. Mardon, personal communication, August 5, 2021). This is her form of counterbalancing the difficulties and strain she faces when helping foster kids and volunteering in bleak situations, such as helping kids that will never mentally mature and be independent.

In addition, couples counselling is quite useful and important, especially for partners with mental illnesses or disorders and their respective spouses. Couples counselling helps pave the way for clearer dialogue and directs it towards meaningful avenues so that problems may be resolved or discussed. But the use of therapy also brings to light an economic standpoint and that certain people from a lower-income background may not have access or availability to use such services which increases the likelihood of a potential breakdown occurring in a person's relationship (Kelly, 2005).

Lastly, Catherine recommends that caregivers or nurses should help patients experiencing mental illness to find something to motivate them and make them want to stay healthy or present and to take their medications, for instance, a hobby, pet, volunteer job, or anything that sustains their interests. It does not matter what the scope or size of this task is, just that it encourages the person. One of the biggest hurdles that many people with mental illness face is taking their meds consistently and for the long-term (C. Mardon, personal communication, August 5, 2021). Without the consistent, long-term use of their meds, those suffering from schizophrenia tend to have a decreased quality of life and a much worse prognosis (C. Mardon, personal communication, August 5, 2021).

Conclusion

This chapter explores schizophrenia, its impacts on both the spouse and support systems (such as caregivers and family), along with the current research looking into the impacts of schizophrenia on spouses of people with schizophrenia. Furthermore, this chapter investigated and contrasted the various relationships that a spouse may have with a partner who has schizophrenia. One such example was Catherine Mardon's relationship with Autsin Mardon, where she shared her personal experience and relationship. The interview with Catherine further sheds light on the unique situation of her relationship with Austin and the perspective of a spouse who has a positive long lasting relationship with a partner who has schizophrenia. Furthermore, the effects of being a spouse to a person with schizophrenia is investigated as well as how caregivers may experience subjective and objective burden. It is noteworthy to mention that Catherine's relationship with Austin is a success story and supports the fact that a positive, stable, long lasting relationship with a person who has schizophrenia is possible. But spouses of an individual with a mental illness have their burdens compounded by stigma and face discrimination wihtin society and even with family. Thus, there must be an increase in awareness and understanding of mental illnesses in order to accept and fully integrate people with mental illness back into society.

CHAPTER 9

The Experience of Families Affected by Schizophrenia

Romina Tabesh

How Schizophrenia Affects Parents and Children

There is no doubt that a parent's well-being affects that of their child. This is the case in children with one or both parents having diagnosed schizophrenia. Interestingly, the more closely related an individual is to someone with schizophrenia, the greater the incidence of that individual being diagnosed with a psychiatric disorder (Hussain, 2020). More specifically, children living with one parent diagnosed with schizophrenia have approximately a 13% chance of developing schizophrenia, whereas those with both parents being clinically diagnosed with the disorder have a 45% chance of developing it (Hussain, 2020). It is therefore important to study the effects of parents with schizophrenia on children as it affects their lifestyle and factors such as their social skills and cognitive development (Hussain, 2020).

The Role of Familial Relations

According to the National Institutes of Health, 10% of children who live with a diagnosed parent with schizophrenia or sibling will also have schizophrenia (Hussain, 2020). These are known as first-order relatives and their connection is an important factor to be considered when examining a child's likelihood of developing schizophrenia. When comparing the effect of first-order relatives with diagnosed schizophrenia to that of second-order relatives— such as grandparents, cousins, aunts or uncles—second-order relatives are shown to have a weaker connection, but still greater than the chances of children in the general population developing the disorder at random (Hussain, 2020). This outlines the uniqueness of children with relatives who have schizophrenia, more specifically who have a parent with schizophrenia.

Adult Children of Parents with Mental Illness

Schizophrenia is a form of 'psychosis' consisting of positive and negative symptoms. Positive symptoms are those which are added to an individual— like hallucinations—and negative symptoms as taking away from an individual—such as the lack of social interest (Hussain, 2020). Living with a parent suffering from schizophrenia may cause debilitating negative impacts on a child (Hussain, 2020). More specifically, the child may begin to developing symptoms of the mental illness (Hussain, 2020). A study done on adult children of a parent with schizophrenia demonstrated this negative impact with regards to the children's measure of resilience. A sample of 45 adult children with one parent diagnosed with schizophrenia were assessed and their experiences were compared to those of children of healthy parents. The study concluded the experiences of these children were distinct, including negative experiences in social and emotional aspects and lack of support from the parent who is ill (Hans et al., 2004). Growing up with a parent with a mental illness can have negative impacts on adult children, but in the presence of a good support system there can be positive effects in terms of developing resilience (Hans et al., 2004).

Children of Parents with Mental Illness

Children of parents diagnosed with mental illness are also affected at a very young age (Duncan & Browning, 2009). In 2009, a study was conducted to answer the question of whether children of parents with mental illness have lower survival rates. Researchers found that children born to women with schizophrenia in particular have a significantly higher risk of child death (Duncan & Browning, 2009). This emphasizes the need to further study and aim to treat parental schizophrenia in order to reduce mortality rates of children exposed to risk during their first 3 years of life (Duncan & Browning, 2009).

Importance of Maternal Schizophrenia

Maternal schizophrenia specifically is known to have an adverse effect on the quality of mother-infant interaction (Manjula & Raguram, 2009). Children of parents with severe mental illness are subject to high risks of poor mental health and social outcomes (Manjula & Raguram, 2009). Hence, children who are raised by a parent diagnosed with schizophrenia may be less likely to attain secure attachment (Manjula & Raguram, 2009). There is a lack of research in the field that explores the needs, experiences, strengths, and vulnerabilities of these children themselves (Manjula & Raguram, 2009). Qualitative methods are therefore required to generate new insights and hypotheses (Manjula & Raguram, 2009). A study was conducted using adults who, as children, were raised by a parent who experienced schizophrenia, revealing a range of attachment problems, resulting in difficulties in forming secure adult relationships (Manjula & Raguram, 2009). Difficulties with trust and intimacy were also found to be common within this group of adult children (Manjula & Raguram, 2009).

Although the precise nature of genetic transmission is still unclear, schizophrenia runs in families. While only 1% of the general population is directly affected by the mental illness, this rises to 10% among the children of parents with schizophrenia (Manjula & Raguram, 2009). There is also evidence that psychosocial factors, such as familial environment, are also involved in the development of schizophrenia (Kuipers 2003). This is of concern, since a child raised by a parent with schizophrenia may face not only genetic risk, but also a poor environment (Leverton 2003).

Postpartum mental illness may have an impact on the child's early development and on secure attachment, resulting in poor social competence and work efficacy in later childhood (Albertsson-Karlgren et al. 2000). Aside from being at a high risk for childhood psychiatric disorders, children raised by parents who suffered from severe mental illness are at a disadvantage as there is reluctance among the parents to seek help for their child's behaviour (Manjula & Raguram, 2009). The parenting capabilities of those who suffer from severe schizophrenia have been a concern, as it affects the child and their development (Manjula & Raguram, 2009).

Maternal mental illness is also associated with fewer responsive behaviours and less positive mother-infant interactions (Manjula & Raguram, 2009). Mothers who are diagnosed with schizophrenia may provide less play stimulation, fewer learning experiences, and less emotional involvement in raising their child, all of which may be associated with poor intellectual and social abilities in children (Goodman, 1987). As a result of this understimulation, these children are more likely to show anxious attachment at about 1 year of age (Manjula & Raguram, 2009).

Effect of Parents with Schizophrenia on Children: Conclusion

It is evident that parents with schizophrenia have a large impact on their children's development. Maternal schizophrenia is of special importance in the case of infants and their need for sufficient stimulation for optimal growth in terms of social and cognitive skills (Manjula & Raguram, 2009). It is also equally important to study the effects of children with schizophrenia on parents. Moreover, in order to better understand the relationship and dynamic between families affected by a mental illness, scientists must also focus on the effects of children with mental illness on their parents.

Parent Caregivers of Children with Schizophrenia

Parent caregivers support the well-being of their adult children with schizophrenia (Young et al., 2019). Due to the extensive amount of care these children need, parent caregivers spend a vast amount of time providing care, which eventually creates changes to their routines, relationships, and overall lifestyle (Young et al., 2019). It is important to study the challenges and changes that schizophrenia brings upon families in order to work towards eliminating such burdens. Schizophrenia affects not only the diagnosed individual, but also their family (Young et al., 2019). Initiating, maintaining, and optimizing treatment across the illness trajectory is a complicated process with numerous challenges for parent caregivers (Young et al., 2019). Parent caregivers are essential in creating a strong support network to improve the mental health, well-being, and aid in achieving the recovery goals of their adult children with schizophrenia (Young et al., 2019). Furthermore, parent caregivers must provide social, physical, emotional, and medical care (Young et al., 2019). They also help with cooking, cleaning, and personal hygiene, as well as administering medication and accompanying the child to and from appointments (Small et al., 2010). Parent caregivers especially provide support in terms of mental health, such as in situations with a child having difficult symptoms such as paranoia (Young et al., 2019).

Responsibilities of Parent Caregivers of Children with Schizophrenia and Their Consequences on Mental Health

Taking into account the numerous and very complex needs of children with schizophrenia, several challenges are imposed on parent caregivers (Young et al., 2019). At the onset of the illness, it is sometimes difficult to identify schizophrenia due to indiscriminate symptoms (Young et al., 2019). As a result, long periods of untreated psychosis sometimes occur, leading to delayed treatment (Yung & Barnaby, 2013). Moreover, untreated psychosis results in more severe symptoms and decreased social and global functioning (Young et al., 2019). During this period of the illness, parent caregivers experience immense guilt and uncertainty (Wiens & Daniluk, 2009). Parent caregivers also struggle to access available and appropriate support such as mental health services during this time (Young et al., 2019).

When adult children diagnosed with schizophrenia are unable to receive the care they require, they are put at risk for frightening symptoms, hospitalization, and even suicide in extreme cases (Higashi et al., 2013). While enduring financial and social costs, family conflict, and poor personal physical and mental health outcomes, parents with a caregiver role of a child with schizophrenia must also learn to navigate illness and service-related challenges (Awad & Voruganti, 2008) . Due to the pressures and stresses imposed on these parent caregivers, anxiety, depression, fear, and anger are frequently reported (Young et al., 2019). They also commonly report physical manifestations such as headaches, stomach pain, constant fatigue, and insomnia (Small et al., 2010). Parent caregivers also report an overall reduction in their quality of life, as well as increased distress due to the difficulty of their role (Sapouna et al., 2013).

In a qualitative study done on the themes of uncertainty, change, and challenges for parent caregivers of adult children diagnosed with schizophrenia, it was found that overall, the parents faced tremendous distress in their lives due to their roles. This was compounded by issues accessing and navigating the healthcare system, as well as interactions with the police (Young et al., 2019). Effective strategies are needed to help parent caregivers cope within their role and gain access to timely and appropriate care (Young et al., 2019).

Conclusion

All in all, it is clear that parent caregivers of children with schizophrenia experience large amounts of stress and anxiety in their lives as a result of their roles (Young et al., 2019). This stress is caused by feelings such as worry and devastation, and fear of not providing enough care for the child. Altogether, these factors contribute to a lower quality of life, worsening mental health and overall well-being. When police intervention is required to initiate treatment, parents require additional support because of the possible implications on their relationships with their adult children with schizophrenia (Young et al., 2019). Interestingly, while current findings resonate with an already abundant area of research concerning difficulties with access to resources in the mental health system, parent caregivers emphasized that the problem was not a shortage of resources, but rather difficulties locating and accessing appropriate services (Young et al., 2019).

The lifetime support needed, along with emotional, social, and financial consequences experienced by individuals with schizophrenia have numerous effects on their families, especially first-order relatives. Familial responses to having a family member with schizophrenia include fear and embarrassment about illness signs and symptoms, care burden, uncertainty about the course of the disease, lack of social support, and stigma (Young et al., 2019). The effects of living with, and caring for a family member affected by schizophrenia may be different depending on the role of the individual within the family. For example, children raised by a parent with schizophrenia are more likely to also develop schizophrenia, and parent caregivers of children with schizophrenia are very likely to experience anxiety due to burden. It is important to continue to provide support and care for individuals affected by mental illness. Research in this field must continue, and authorities such as the police need further, more extensive training in order to better interact with, and help, individuals with mental illnesses such as schizophrenia. It is very important for affected families to come together and to seek help, and for resources to become more easily accessible to such families. Researchers must continue their work in order to progress towards an effective treatment for people affected by mental illness including schizophrenia.

References

CHAPTER 1

Jablensky, A. (2010). The diagnostic concept of schizophrenia: Its history, evolution, and future prospects. Schizophrenia, 12(3), 271–287. https://doi. org/10.31887/dcns.2010.12.3/ajablensky

Brisch, R., Saniotis, A., Wolf, R., Bielau, H., Bernstein, H.-G., Steiner, J., Bogerts, B., Braun, K., Jankowski, Z., Kumaratilake, J., Henneberg, M., & Gos, T. (2014). Corrigendum: The role of dopamine in schizophrenia from a NEURO-BIOLOGICAL and evolutionary PERSPECTIVE: Old fashioned, but still in vogue. Frontiers in Psychiatry, 5. https://doi.org/10.3389/fpsyt.2014.00110

Li, P., L. Snyder, G., & E. Vanover, K. (2016). Dopamine targeting drugs for the treatment of schizophrenia: Past, present and future. Current Topics in Medicinal Chemistry, 16(29), 3385–3403. https://doi.org/10.2174/1568026 616666160608084834

Patel, K. R., Cherian, J., Gohil, K., & Atkinson, D. (2014). Schizophrenia: overview and treatment options. P & T : a peer-reviewed journal for formulary management, 39(9), 638–645.

Altschuler E. L. (2001). One of the oldest cases of schizophrenia in Gogol's Diary of a Madman. BMJ (Clinical research ed.), 323(7327), 1475–1477. https://doi. org/10.1136/bmj.323.7327.1475

Lavretsky , H., Mueser, K. T., & Jeste, D. V. (2008). Clinical handbook of schizo-phrenia . Guilford Press.

Jones, K. (2000). Insulin coma therapy in schizophrenia. Journal of the Royal Society of Medicine, 93(3), 147–149. https://doi.org/10.1177/014107680009300313

Berrios, G. E. (1997). The origins of psychosurgery: Shaw, burckhardt and Moniz. History of

Psychiatry, 8(29), 061–81. https://doi.org/10.1177/0957154x9700802905

CHAPTER 2

Bassett, A. S., Collins, E. J., Nuttall, S. E., & Honer, W. G. (1993). Positive and negative symptoms in families with schizophrenia. Schizophrenia Research, 11(1).https://doi.org/10.1016/0920-9964(93)90033-F

Carpenter, W. T., & Koenig, J. I. (2008). The evolution of drug development in schizophrenia: Past issues and future opportunities. In Neuropsychopharmacology (Vol. 33, Issue 9).https://doi.org/10.1038/sj.npp.1301639

Dobber, J., Latour, C., de Haan, L., Scholte op Reimer, W., Peters, R., Barkhof, E., & van Meijel B.(2018). Medication adherence in patients with schizophrenia: A qualitative study of the patient process in motivational interviewing. BMC Psychiatry, 18(1).   https://doi.org/10.1186/s12888-018-1724-9

Frese, F. J., Knight, E. L., & Saks, E. (2009). Recovery from schizophrenia: With views of   psychiatrists, psychologists, and others diagnosed with this disorder. Schizophrenia Bulletin, 35(2). https://doi.org/10.1093/schbul/sbn175

George, M., Maheshwari, S., Chandran, S., Manohar, J. S., & Sathyanarayana Rao, T. S. (2017).   Understanding the schizophrenia prodrome. Indian Journal of Psychiatry, 59(4).   https://doi.org/10.4103/psychiatry.IndianJPsychiatry_464_17

Mardon, A. (2021, August 04). Personal communication [Personal interview].

Trifu, S. C., Vlăduți, A., & Trifu, A. I. (2020). Genetic aspects in schizophrenia. Receptoraltheories. metabolic theories. In Romanian Journal of Morphology and Embryology (Vol. 61, Issue 1). https://doi.org/10.47162/RJME.61.1.03

CHAPTER 3

Andreasen, N. C., & Flaum, M. (1991). Schizophrenia: The characteristic symptoms. Schizophrenia Bulletin, 17(1), 27–49. https://doi.org/10.1093/schbul/17.1.27

Cachope, R., & Cheer, J. F. (2014). Local control of striatal dopamine release. Frontiers in Behavioral Neuroscience, 8. https://doi.org/10.3389/fnbeh.2014.00188

Egerton, A., Grace, A. A., Stone, J., Bossong, M. G., Sand, M., & McGuire, P. (2020). Glutamate in schizophrenia: Neurodevelopmental perspectives and drug development. Schizophrenia Research, 223, 59–70. https://doi.org/10.1016/j.schres.2020.09.013

Hancock, S. D., & McKim, W. A. (2018). Neurophysiology, Neurotransmitters, and the Nervous System. In Drugs and behavior: An introduction to behavioral pharmacology (7th ed., pp. 50–84). essay, Pearson.

Howes, O. D., & Murray, R. M. (2014). Schizophrenia: An integrated sociodevelopmental-cognitive model. The Lancet, 383(9929), 1677–1687. https://doi.org/10.1016/s0140-6736(13)62036-x

McCutcheon, R. A., Krystal, J. H., & Howes, O. D. (2020). Dopamine and glutamate in schizophrenia: Biology, symptoms and treatment. World Psychiatry, 19(1), 15–33. https://doi.org/10.1002/wps.20693

Meyer, J. S., & Quenzer, L. F. (2019). Schizophrenia: Antipsychotic Drugs. In Drugs, the brain and behavior (3rd ed., pp. 633–671). essay, Oxford University Press.

Robertson, D. M., & Dinsdale, H. B. (1972). The nervous system . Williams & Wilkins.

CHAPTER 4

Dein, S. (2017). Recent work on culture and schizophrenia: Epidemiological and anthropological approaches. Global Journal Of Archaeology & Anthropology, 1(3), 64-67. doi: 10.19080/gjaa.2017.01.555562

Essock, S. M. (2017). When social and environmental adversity causes schizophrenia. The American Journal of Psychiatry, 174(2), 89.

Fearon, P., & Morgan, C. (2006). Environmental factors in schizophrenia: The role of migrant studies. Schizophrenia Bulletin, 32(3), 405–407. https://doi.org/10.1093/schbul/sbj076

Habel, U., Gur, R. C., Mandal, M. K., Salloum, J. B., Gur, R. E., & Schneider, F. (2000). Emotional processing in schizophrenia across cultures: Standardized measures of discrimination and experience. Schizophrenia Research, 42(1), 57-58. https://doi.org/10.1016/S0920-9964(99)00093-6

Hooley, J. M. (2010). Social factors in schizophrenia. Current Directions in Psychological Science: A Journal of the American Psychological Society, 19(4), 238–240. https://doi.org/10.1177/0963721410377597

Krabbendam, L., & Van Os, J. (2005). Schizophrenia and urbanicity: A major environmental influence - Conditional on genetic risk. Schizophrenia Bulletin, 31(4), 795–797. https://doi.org/10.1093/schbul/sbi060

Myers, N. L. (2011). Update: Schizophrenia across cultures. Current Psychiatry Reports, 13(4), 305–308. https://doi.org/10.1007/s11920-011-0208-0

van Os, J., & McGuffin, P. (2003). Can the social environment cause schizophrenia? British Journal of Psychiatry, 182(4), 291–292. https://doi.org/10.1192/bjp.182.4.291

CHAPTER 5

Arnold, S. E., Lee, V. M., Gur, R. E., & Trojanowski, J. Q. (1991). Abnormal expression of two microtubule-associated proteins (MAP2 and MAP5) in specific subfields of the hippocampal formation in schizophrenia. Proceedings of the National Academy of Sciences of the United States of America, 88(23), 10850–10854. https://doi.org/10.1073/pnas.88.23.10850

Giersch, A., & Mishara, A. L. (2017). Is Schizophrenia a Disorder of Consciousness? Experimental and Phenomenological Support for Anomalous Unconscious Processing. Frontiers in Psychology, 8(1659). doi:10.3389/fpsyg.2017.01659

Haenschel, C., Bittner, R. A., Waltz, J., Haertling, F., Wibral, M., Singer, W., ... Rodriguez, E. (2009). Cortical Oscillatory Activity Is Critical for Working Memory as Revealed by Deficits in Early-Onset Schizophrenia. Journal of Neuroscience, 29(30), 9481–9489. doi:10.1523/jneurosci.1428-09.2009

Hameroff, S., & Penrose, R. (2014). Consciousness in the universe. Physics of Life Reviews, 11(1), 39–78. doi:10.1016/j.plrev.2013.08.002

Lopes da Silva F. (2013). EEG and MEG: relevance to neuroscience. Neuron, 80(5), 1112–1128. https://doi.org/10.1016/j.neuron.2013.10.017

Musall, S., von Pföstl, V., Rauch, A., Logothetis, N. K., & Whittingstall, K. (2012). Effects of Neural Synchrony on Surface EEG. Cerebral Cortex, 24(4), 1045–1053. doi:10.1093/cercor/bhs389

Rodriguez, E., George, N., Lachaux, J.-P., Martinerie, J., Renault, B., & Varela, F. J. (1999). Perception's shadow: long-distance synchronization of human brain activity. Nature, 397(6718), 430–433. doi:10.1038/17120

Shin, Y. W., O'Donnell, B. F., Youn, S., & Kwon, J. S. (2011). Gamma oscillation in schizophrenia. Psychiatry investigation, 8(4), 288–296. https://doi.org/10.4306/pi.2011.8.4.288

Uhlhaas, P. J., & Singer, W. (2010). Abnormal neural oscillations and synchrony in schizophrenia. Nature Reviews Neuroscience, 11(2), 100–113. doi:10.1038/nrn2774

Venkatasubramanian G. (2015). Understanding schizophrenia as a disorder of consciousness: biological correlates and translational implications from quantum theory perspectives. Clinical psychopharmacology and neuroscience : the official scientific journal of the Korean College of Neuropsychopharmacology, 13(1), 36–47. https://doi.org/10.9758/cpn.2015.13.1.36

Ward, L. M. (2003). Synchronous neural oscillations and cognitive processes. Trends in Cognitive Sciences, 7(12), 553–559. doi:10.1016/j.tics.2003.10.012

Williams, S., & Boksa, P. (2010). Gamma oscillations and schizophrenia. Journal of Psychiatry & Neuroscience, 35(2), 75–77. https://doi.org/10.1503/jpn.100021

Williams, L. M., Whitford, T. J., Nagy, M., Flynn, G., Harris, A. W., Silverstein, S. M., & Gordon, E. (2009). Emotion-elicited gamma synchrony in patients with first-episode schizophrenia: a neural correlate of social cognition outcomes. Journal of Psychiatry & Neuroscience, 34(4), 303–313.

CHAPTER 6

González-Torres, M. A., Oraa, R., Arístegui, M., Fernández-Rivas, A., & Guimon, J. (2006).

Stigma and discrimination towards people with schizophrenia and their family members. Social Psychiatry and Psychiatric Epidemiology, 42(1), 14–23. https://doi.org/10.1007/s00127-006-0126-3

Insel, T. R. (2010). Rethinking schizophrenia. Nature, 468(7321), 187–193.

https://doi.org/10.1038/nature09552

Larson, M. K., Walker, E. F., & Compton, M. T. (2010). Early signs, diagnosis and therapeutics

of the prodromal phase of schizophrenia and related psychotic disorders. Expert Review of Neurotherapeutics, 10(8), 1347–1359. https://doi.org/10.1586/ern.10.93

Mcglashan, T. H., & Woods, S. (2011, March 15). Early antecedents and detection of

schizophrenia. Psychiatric Times. https://www.psychiatrictimes.com/view/early-antecedents-and-detection-schizophrenia.

Stuart H. (2003). Violence and mental illness: an overview. World psychiatry : official journal of

the World Psychiatric Association (WPA), 2(2), 121–124.

Vala, V. D. (2021, August 7). Dr. Austin Mardon: Prodrome and Antecedents of Schizophrenia.

personal.

Welham, J., Isohanni, M., Jones, P., & McGrath, J. (2009). The antecedents of Schizophrenia: A

review of birth cohort studies. Schizophrenia Bulletin, 35(3), 603–623. https://doi.org/10.1093/schbul/sbn084

CHAPTER 7

Addington, J., Piskulic, D., & Marshall, C. (2010). Psychosocial treatments for schizophrenia. Current Directions in Psychological Science, 19(4), 260–263. https://doi.org/10.1177/0963721410377743

Meltzer, H. Y. (1997). Treatment-resistant schizophrenia - the role of clozapine. Current Medical Research and Opinion, 14(1), 1–20. https://doi.org/10.1185/03007999709113338

Patel, K. R., Jessica Cherian, J., Gohil, K., & Atkinson, D. (2014). Schizophrenia: Overview and treatment options. P&T, 39(9), 638–645.

Vanasse, A., Blais, L., Courteau, J., Cohen, A. A., Roberge, P., Larouche, A., Grignon, S., Fleury, M.-J., Lesage, A., Demers, M.-F., Roy, M.-A., Carrier, J.-D., & Delorme, A. (2016). Comparative effectiveness and safety of antipsychotic drugs in schizophrenia treatment: A real-world observational study. Acta Psychiatrica Scandinavica, 134(5), 374–384. https://doi.org/10.1111/acps.12621

CHAPTER 8

Jungbauer, J., Wittmund, B., Dietrich, S., & Angermeyer, M. C. (2004). The Disregarded

Caregivers: Subjective Burden in Spouses of Schizophrenia Patients.

Schizophrenia Bulletin, 30(3), 665–675. https://doi.org/10.1093/oxfordjournals. schb ul.a007114

Kahn, R. S., Sommer, I. E.,, Murray, R., Myder-Lindenber, A., Weinberger, A. R., Cannon, T.,

O'Donovan, M., Correll, C., Kane, J. M., Os, J. V., & Insel, T. R. (2015). Schizophrenia.

Nature Reviews Disease Primers, 1(15067). 0.1038/nrdp.2015.67

Kelly, B. D. (2005). Structural violence and schizophrenia. Soc Sci Med, 61, 721-730. https://rea

der.elsevier.com/reader/sd/pii/S0277953605000195?token=14D0117DBBDAB-0D5C237CFC264218DF756EF6AB4EF98C9C3B683435482064A764C32 E61E3E5819073D08B2B1E8066A4F&originRegion=us-east-1&originCreation=20210816042623

Kumari, S., Singh, A. R., Verma, A. N., Verma, P. k., & Chaudhury, S. (2009). Subjective burden

on spouses of schizophrenia patients. Ind Psychiatry J, 18(2), 97-100. 10.4103/0972-674 8.62268

CHAPTER 9

Duncan, G., & Browning, J. (2009). Adult attachment in children raised by parents with schizophrenia. Journal of Adult Development, 16(2), 76–86. https://doi.org/10.1007/s10804-009-9054-2

Hans, S. L., Auerbach, J. G., Styr, B., & Marcus, J. (2004). Offspring of parents with schizophrenia: Mental disorders during childhood and adolescence. Schizophrenia Bulletin, 30(2), 303–315. https://doi.org/10.1093/oxfordjournals.schbul.a007080

Herbert, H. S., Manjula, M., & Philip, M. (2013). Growing up with a parent having schizophrenia: Experiences and resilience in the offsprings. Indian Journal of Psychological Medicine, 35(2), 148. https://doi.org/10.4103/0253-7176.116243

Hussain, S. (2020). The impacts of parental schizophrenia on the psychosocial well-being of offspring: A systematic review. Quality of Life - Biopsychosocial Perspectives. https://doi.org/10.5772/intechopen.91658

Liu, T.-C., Chen, C.-S., & Loh, C. P. (2010). Do children of parents with mental illness have lower survival rate? A population-based study. Comprehensive Psychiatry, 51(3), 250–255. https://doi.org/10.1016/j.comppsych.2009.07.004

Manjula, M., & Raguram, A. (2009). Self-concept in adult children of schizophrenic parents: An exploratory study. International Journal of Social Psychiatry, 55(5), 471–479. https://doi.org/10.1177/0020764008094732

Young, L., Digel Vandyk, A., Daniel Jacob, J., McPherson, C., & Murata, L. (2019). Being parent caregivers for adult children with schizophrenia. Issues in Mental Health Nursing, 40(4), 297–303. https://doi.org/10.1080/01612840.2018.1524531

www.ingramcontent.com/pod-product-compliance
Lightning Source LLC
Chambersburg PA
CBHW071750270326
41928CB00013B/2869